A STUDENT'S GUIDE TO ASSESSMENT AND DIAGNOSIS USING THE ICD-10-CM

A STUDENT'S GUIDE TO ASSESSMENT AND DIAGNOSIS USING THE ICD-10-CM

PSYCHOLOGICAL AND BEHAVIORAL CONDITIONS

JACK SCHAFFER and EMIL RODOLFA

American Psychological Association • Washington, DC

Published by
American Psychological Association
750 First Street, NE
Washington, DC 20002-4242
www.apa.org

To order
APA Order Department
P.O. Box 92984
Washington, DC 20090-2984
Tel: (800) 374-2721; Direct: (202) 336-5510
Fax: (202) 336-5502; TDD/TTY: (202) 336-6123
Online: www.apa.org/pubs/books/
E-mail: order@apa.org

In the U.K., Europe, Africa, and the Middle East, copies may be ordered from
American Psychological Association
3 Henrietta Street
Covent Garden, London
WC2E 8LU England

Typeset in Meridien by Circle Graphics, Inc., Columbia, MD

Printer: Sheridan Books, Ann Arbor, MI
Cover Designer: Mercury Publishing Services, Rockville, MD

The opinions and statements published are the responsibility of the authors, and such opinions and statements do not necessarily represent the policies of the American Psychological Association.

Library of Congress Cataloging-in-Publication Data

Schaffer, Jack.
  A student's guide to assessment and diagnosis using the ICD-10-CM : psychological and behavioral conditions / Jack Schaffer and Emil Rodolfa.
    pages cm
  Includes bibliographical references and index.
  ISBN 978-1-4338-2093-9 — ISBN 1-4338-2093-5 1. Mental illness—Classification. 2. Mental illness—Diagnosis—Problems, exercises, etc. I. Rodolfa, Emil. II. Title.
  RC455.2.C4S33 2016
  616.89'075—dc23
                              2015018198

British Library Cataloguing-in-Publication Data
A CIP record is available from the British Library.

Printed in the United States of America
First Edition

http://dx.doi.org/10.1037/14778-000

To my family—Jan, Josh, Alethea,
and their children—Sophia, Soleil, Solomon, and Aurora
—Jack Schaffer

And to mine—Mary Jo, Kit, and Joie
—Emil Rodolfa

Contents

Acknowledgments

Writing a book is a formidable task. Many psychologists have written more than one book, and some have written dozens. We are in awe! This project would not have been possible without the support, assistance, and input of many people. To a very large degree, what follows in this text is based on the authors' 30-plus years of experience, in which numerous graduate school faculty; practicum, internship, and post doc supervisors; colleagues and mentors; and students have played an important role. In that list, a number of colleagues deserve special mention.

For me (Jack Schaffer), at the top of that list is the late Richard Friberg, PhD, a licensed psychologist with whom I consulted regularly for more than 30 years. What I learned from him about how one approaches the assessment process cannot be overemphasized. And, he became a dear friend in the process. A second person who deserves special mention is Tom Boll, PhD. During my internship I spent a few days with Tom at his clinic in Charlottesville, Virginia, and in that brief time, followed by reading much of what he has written about assessment, I got started in the direction my assessment career took over the next 35 years. Much of what is written in Chapter 2 is thanks to the perspectives and insights provided by Dick and Tom. Beyond those two, however, is a long list of colleagues who have influenced me, guided me, taught me, and sometimes, protected me from myself. To all of my supportive colleagues, I am deeply appreciative. And, of course, to my wife, Jan, without whose support and occasional chiding I would not be the person I am today.

I (Emil Rodolfa) thank so many colleagues who have influenced my professional practice of psychology. There are truly too many colleagues and friends to mention. But I would be remiss if I did not thank Robert Reilley, PhD, my major professor, academic advisor, dissertation chair, mentor, and friend, who taught me not only how to practice psychology but also how to be a psychologist. I appreciate all that he taught me (and tried to teach me) and all that I learned from him. I also thank my wife, Mary Jo, who has greatly supported all my professional endeavors. We have had a great ride together. Thanks for the memories.

We also thank the following people who reviewed and provided feedback on parts of this manuscript: Tom Boll, PhD; Gary Fischler, PhD; David Fisher, PhD; Floyd Jennings, JD, PhD; and Dan Tranel, PhD. In some cases, we adopted what they suggested, because we thought them correct. In other instances, we ignored their advice because we liked what we had said better. Ultimately, you the reader will have to decide how useful our writing is.

A special word of thanks also goes to a number of individuals at the American Psychological Association: to Gary VandenBos and Julia Frank-McNeil, who asked us to commit a few words to paper; to Claude Conyers, whose gentle prodding and encouragement was greatly appreciated and truly helped us get started; and to David Becker and Lynn Bufka, who thoughtfully reviewed and edited our work, and to Nikki Seifert, our copyeditor, whose attention to detail helped us improve the clarity of our message. Each one of the terrific staff at APA Books helped us produce a work that we hope will be helpful to you.

Jack Schaffer also thanks Emil Rodolfa. We have become collaborators on a variety of projects, mutual motivators, and, close friends. Emil Rodolfa also thanks Jack Schaffer. Working on this project was hard work and time consuming (more time consuming than I ever would have imagined), yet enjoyable because of that mutual motivation, encouragement, and friendship.

A STUDENT'S GUIDE TO ASSESSMENT AND DIAGNOSIS USING THE ICD-10-CM

PSYCHOLOGICAL AND BEHAVIORAL CONDITIONS

JACK SCHAFFER and EMIL RODOLFA

American Psychological Association • Washington, DC

Introduction

This book is part of a series of books published by the American Psychological Association (APA) on the classification system known as the *International Statistical Classification of Diseases and Related Health Problems* (ICD) developed by the World Health Organization (WHO). As we describe in more detail in Chapter 1, the ICD has been the standard in medical classification internationally since the mid-19th century. It is now in its 10th edition (ICD–10; WHO, 2016), with the 11th edition scheduled for dissemination by the WHO sometime in 2017. As we discuss the ICD–10, if you have interest in learning about some projected changes and the development of the ICD–11, see Tyrer et al. (2011).

The ICD–10 was endorsed by the WHO in 1990 and adopted for use in most countries in the world by 1994 (WHO, 2016). The WHO allows each country to adapt the ICD for its own specific clinical needs. In the United States, that adaptation is referred to as the Clinical Modification, hence, the ICD–10–CM (National Center for Health Statistics, 2015).

http://dx.doi.org/10.1037/14778-001
A Student's Guide to Assessment and Diagnosis Using the ICD–10–CM: Psychological and Behavioral Conditions, by J. Schaffer and E. Rodolfa

On October 1, 2015, the United States switched from using the ICD–9 to using the ICD–10 because the limitations of the ICD–9, primarily in the number of diagnostic categories present, were becoming increasingly obvious and problematic. Although the ICD is fundamentally a list of causes of death, expanded to include morbidity, it is recognized that not all health-related problems fit into those two categories, so the ICD–10–CM incorporates the flexibility to include a variety of signs and symptoms that would end up in a patient's chart and about which gathering of health information could be of benefit. At the same time, unless the number of categories is limited, the system is not very helpful, so the ICD–10–CM provides a balance between comprehensiveness and practicality. The goal of the ICD endeavor has been to provide a specific category for any condition that either has importance to the well-being of the population or occurs with some frequency.

In addition, unbeknownst to many or most psychologists, it is not the *Diagnostic and Statistical Manual of Mental Disorders* (*DSM*) of the American Psychiatric Association (e.g., 2013) that is the standard classification system used by agencies of the U.S. government (e.g., Medicare, Medicaid) and by most private insurance companies—it is the ICD (specifically, ICD–9–CM until October 1, 2015, and ICD–10–CM starting on October 1, 2015). The change from ICD–9–CM to ICD–10–CM constituted a significant change in codes, as we describe in Chapter 1. Briefly stated, the codes used by the fourth edition of the *DSM* (American Psychiatric Association, 1994) and the ICD–9–CM were virtually identical. The development of the fifth edition of the *DSM* (American Psychiatric Association, 2013) led to some divergence in codes (i.e., the numbering system used to refer to specific diagnoses) and with the ICD–10–CM, the divergence has increased.

Thus, this series of books published by APA is intended to educate mental health professionals, psychologists in particular, in the use of the ICD system, specifically, the ICD–10–CM. The goal is to help mental health professionals understand the requirements for billing insurance companies under the ICD–10–CM and to assist them to become more consistent in their thinking and diagnostic procedures with an increasingly globalized psychology.

Welcome to Our World

This book, focused on the ICD–10–CM, is written primarily for graduate students and interns in psychology. Our specific goal is to assist in their preparation for the diagnostic tasks they will encounter as practicing psychologists in the very near future. In other words, this book has been written to help students think like psychologists, including using critical thinking skills, and learn to use and apply the classification system of the ICD–10. However, we firmly believe that diagnosis is part of a broader enterprise for psychologists that includes, centrally, the assessment of the personality, social context, needs, problems, and strengths of the individuals with whom they work. Therefore, this book focuses to a large degree on assessment, placing the ICD–10–CM diagnostic system at the center of that assessment process.

To that end, the book comprises 10 chapters, in addition to this brief introduction. Chapter 1 presents a primer of the ICD–10–CM system, with the goal of providing the historical context for the ICD system and, more important, the specific steps one must take to arrive at the correct diagnostic code using the ICD–10–CM system.

Chapters 2 and 3 explore assessment and diagnosis and provide an overview of the numerous issues a psychologist should consider in the process of assessing an individual and arriving at a diagnosis. For the experienced psychologist, assessment of a person is an endlessly interesting and challenging process. The goal is, in the matter of a few short hours and with a limited number of psychological tools, to come to an understanding of a person, such that the goals of the assessment can be accomplished, whether the goals have to do with, for example, the provision of psychotherapy and the resolution of some problem; or the development of an assessment process resulting in a report to a court, as happens in forensic psychology; or responding to another professional who makes a referral. It is the complexity of trying to understand a complicated human being that makes the process interesting and challenging, even for the experienced psychologist. That complexity can be daunting to a student. Chapters 3 is our attempt to provide an outline of the process and some of the challenges of undertaking such a formidable task as trying to understand another human being. Obviously, these two chapters cannot provide everything that a student can and should know about assessment. Hence, supplemental resources that might be helpful are provided in Chapter 10. Chapters 2 and 3, however, provide a philosophical perspective regarding psychological assessment leading to the process of diagnosis, which requires knowledge and skill to carry it out in an appropriate and competent manner.

The remainder of the book relies on Chapters 4, 5, and 6 as its core. Each of these three chapters provides a case that serves as a basis for discussion of issues involved in the assessment process. These three cases, chosen in part with commonly used ICD–10–CM diagnostic categories in mind and in part on the clinical experiences of the two authors, cover three very different clinical situations. The first case, described in Chapter 4, is a referral to a graduate student clinic for assessment as part of a treatment process, and provides a consideration of issues related to students providing psychological services. The second, described in Chapter 5, is a referral for an assessment in a medical setting, with the possibility of treatment follow-up. What is different from the first case, but common in the real world, is that very few specifics are provided with the referral, creating a challenge to know what should be done and how. The third case, described in Chapter 6, is a referral by an attorney. This referral has a very complex social history and presents with very challenging psychological issues. The referral is for an assessment without the potential for follow-up treatment. These three cases were conceived with the goal of providing a range of problems and situations that are typically seen in clinical practice. After describing each case, we discuss the process a psychologist undertakes in thinking about clinical cases, both in terms of how one approaches the assessment process, that is, what assessment methods to use and what type of data to collect, and subsequently how those collected data influence the diagnostic decisions and differential diagnoses using the ICD–10–CM.

Chapters 7 through 9 all have as their core the three cases. In these chapters, we ask readers to continue to apply their critical thinking skills to the information presented, skills that we believe are central to the competent practice of psychology. (More on the important issue of critical thinking momentarily.)

Chapter 7 examines how ethical issues are incorporated into professional practice. It begins with a general presentation on ethical standards and then considers the ethical issues raised by each of the three cases.

Chapter 8 presents a discussion of risk, that is, how one approaches clinical practice in a way that minimizes risk to the practitioner. Again, after some general comments about risk management, we consider the potential risks in each of the three cases, along with methods for minimizing those risks and thereby maximizing the positive outcomes for both patient and psychologist.

Chapter 9 covers disposition, that is, how one responds to a given case to reach whatever goals are set. With the first case, we present a possible treatment plan that could be developed, given the data available in that case. Case 2 is primarily an assessment case, but treatment issues are also examined. Case 3 is strictly an assessment case, so the focus of the discussion is on how to approach a case with such limits.

Chapter 10 is a snapshot of resources for the new psychologist. We have relied on many of these resources during our careers; many are classics with updated editions, and all are useful books or websites that exist to provide guidance in the practice of psychology. This chapter describes resources for the following areas, as well as a comment about additional resources: ICD, diagnosis, assessment, interviewing, practice guidelines, evidence-based practice, ethics, risk management.

Critical Thinking

We are certain that as you matriculated into your academic program, you heard comments from your faculty about the importance of critical thinking. But what is critical thinking?

The numerous definitions of *critical thinking* (Brookfield, 1987; Clayton, 2007; Facione, 2013; Scriven & Paul, 1987) all stress the need for the thinker (i.e., you) not to take things at face value but to examine systematically and thoroughly all of the information you have, challenge your conceptualizations of this information, and then draw conclusions in a self-disciplined and self-examining manner. We discuss this process and additional reasons for using critical thinking throughout this text.

Clearly, critical thinking is essential to the practice of psychology, as the Association of State and Provincial Psychology Boards (ASPPB) has incorporated this concept into its framework of Competencies Expected of Psychologists at the Point of Licensure (ASPPB, 2014a; Rodolfa et al., 2013). ASPPB lists three competencies that specifically include the concepts of critical thinking specific to the practice of psychology:

1. Select relevant research literature and critically review its assumptions, conceptualization, methodology, interpretation, and generalizability.
2. Interpret, evaluate, and integrate results of data-collection activities within the context of scientific/professional knowledge to formulate and reformulate working hypotheses, conceptualizations, and recommendations.
3. Articulate a rationale for decisions and psychological services that rely on objective supporting data (e.g., research results, base rates, epidemiological data).

You will see, as you move through the process to become a licensed psychologist, that licensing boards will require that you are able to think critically about your work as a psychologist. It is also important to note that the academic associations in psychology have worked together to develop models of competency, as well as the entity in psychology that accredits training programs. All of these competency models acknowledge the importance of critical thinking in the development of psychological competencies and the functioning of the psychologist.

As you can see from this discussion, we believe, and the profession emphasizes, that critical thinking is essential to the work of a psychologist. This book is written to help you do just that.

What's in a Name?

Before we conclude this chapter, we believe it is important to briefly discuss three issues. The first is our choice to use the term *patients* instead of *clients*. Psychology does not have a universally accepted term to refer to the individuals to whom we provide psychological services. *Patient* is the term most commonly used in medical settings, but it has the disadvantage of implying a hierarchical relationship. *Client* is the term most used in university counseling clinics, but it comes originally from business settings and has the disadvantage of implying a professional relationship in which the therapist provides information and advice as an accountant or attorney might, rather than a caring relationship in which the therapist treats mental disorders. We do not have an ideal term for a person with some psychological issues who is looking for a provider with expertise in listening and helping the person explore various behavioral and cognitive options, as well as teaching the person new behavioral and cognitive skills to treat psychological problems. As a result, we have chosen to use the term *patient*, partly because this text focuses on the issue of clinical assessment and diagnosis, and partly because we believe the term *patient* more accurately captures the relationship between psychologist and the individual seeking service. But it was a close call. We do, however, use the term *client* to refer to recipients of psychological services who are not individuals, such as couples, families, or organizations.

The second issue is how a patient is addressed, that is, by first name or more formally. We have chosen to refer to Lynn (Case 1; see Chapter 4) by her first name and John Smith (Case 2; see Chapter 5) and Anne Sanchez (Case 3; see Chapter 6) more formally, for several reasons. First, which form of address is most appropriate is in part a function of setting. The case of Lynn came from a university setting where most of the recipients of psychological services are students and typically they are addressed by their first name and use of a more formal address would seem awkward, at best, and distancing, at worst.

In other settings, such as medical or forensic settings, from which Cases 2 and 3 come, the use of formal address is much more common. In addition, in medical settings, most physicians and psychologists are referred to only as "Dr." For a medical or psychological provider in turn to refer to his or her patient by first name appears to us to be disrespectful, as it stresses the inequality of the relationship. When discussing the case of Anne Sanchez, we also use a more formal address due to the setting and referral source, an attorney, where formality also helps define the nature of the professional relationship and boundaries.

We are raising this issue and suggesting that the use of address is important because it has to do with the context and the nature of the professional relationship. How you address your patients should be carefully considered and discussed directly with them. We chose to use both means of address to raise this issue and indicate that both should be considered.

Third, throughout this book, we use the terms *diagnosis* and *assessment* repeatedly. Although similar, they are not the same thing. *Diagnosis* has to do with choosing a specific category to apply to a person. In this text, we use the ICD–10–CM classification system for that purpose. An *assessment* is the process of understanding the issues and problems of the person in the role of patient. One uses the assessment process to arrive at a diagnosis, and vice versa. This distinction is discussed in more detail in Chapters 2 and 3.

A further distinction relevant to our book is that between descriptive and dynamic diagnosis (Oyebode, 2008). *Descriptive* diagnosis, the approach used by the ICD–10–CM, focuses on a statement of what is, that is, classifies individuals on the basis of the signs and symptoms they presented, that is, the behaviors, cognitions, and emotions present in the person. *Dynamic* diagnosis attempts to explain why those symptoms are present, usually using a behavioral, cognitive, or affective theory to explain the underlying causes of the symptoms. In this book, we attempt to describe rather than explain—that is, we describe the processes necessary to understand who the patient is; what experiences, objective and subjective, the person has; how the person presents to others; and whether those experiences and behaviors are in some way abnormal. We do not try to explain the underlying causes of such behaviors. That would be a different task for a different text.

In closing, we hope that this text contributes to your understanding of the ICD–10–CM; enhances your ability to assess, diagnose, and consider dispositions for your patients; enriches your capacity to think like a psychologist; and provide you a foundation to take the next step and put your knowledge into practice under close supervision.

Note to Instructors

This book is intended primarily for use in graduate training, in particular, in courses on assessment and psychopathology. It focuses on the issues involved in engaging in a process of psychological assessment, and it describes how one can use a diagnostic system, such as the ICD–10–CM, to arrive at a better diagnostic understanding of the patient, hence its usefulness in a course on psychopathology. We are in the process of developing a casebook as a companion text, which is included in the APA series on the ICD–10–CM. This casebook will help students examine 16 diagnostic categories using the framework provided in this current text. We anticipate that it will be available in 2016.

The ICD–10
A Primer

1

T he *International Statistical Classification of Diseases and Related Health Problems* (ICD) is a compendium of diseases and causes of death created by the World Health Organization (WHO, 2016), an agency of the United Nations that is charged with overseeing and promoting public health internationally. As part of this overall mission, the WHO developed the ICD, now in its 10th edition (ICD–10), to track and interpret causes of death and illnesses throughout the world.

The ICD has become the international standard system for diagnosing and reporting illnesses. In the United States, it has been the system used by physicians for diagnosing physical illnesses and causes of death and by private insurance companies, Medicare, and Medicaid for reimbursing practicing health care professionals.

http://dx.doi.org/10.1037/14778-002
A Student's Guide to Assessment and Diagnosis Using the ICD–10–CM: Psychological and Behavioral Conditions, by J. Schaffer and E. Rodolfa

A Brief History of the ICD

At its first meeting in Brussels in 1853, the International Statistical Congress directed the development of a list of causes of death, which it adopted at its next meeting in 1855 and further revised at four subsequent meetings. Its successor organization, the International Statistical Institute, meeting in Vienna in 1891, formed a committee whose charge was to continue this work by developing a universally acceptable classification system for the causes of death. Thus was born the initial international classification system, based largely on the system used by the city of Paris, which in turn was based on a synthesis of systems used in England, Germany, and Switzerland. Seeing its utility, a number of cities and countries in Europe and South America adopted this classification system. In 1898, the American Public Health Association recommended its adoption for use in Canada, Mexico, and the United States, with an additional recommendation that it be revised every 10 years to reflect changes in both knowledge and terminology (ICD, Vol. 2). Subsequent international conferences were convened to create such revisions in 1900, 1909, 1920, 1929, and 1938. It was at the Fifth International Conference in 1938 that the need for a corresponding list of the comprehensive causes of diseases, whether or not fatal, was recognized and the list's development directed.

This initiative used as its starting point a study conducted by the U.S. government in 1929 on methods of selecting the main causes of death. The U.S. government responded in 1945 by the Secretary of State appointing members to a newly formed U.S. Committee on Joint Causes of Death. This committee started with the assumption that it needed to consider not only diseases that resulted in mortality but also the morbidity of the diseases, that is, the degree to which a disease initiates or contributes to a series of medical events that can result in death or impairment.

The WHO, founded in 1948 as a specialized agency of the newly created United Nations, was formed to promote world health. One of its first actions was to help plan and to participate in the Sixth Decennial Revision Conference to update the *International List of Causes of Death*, in particular in light of work of the Committee on Joint Causes of Diseases, the American committee convened in 1945. The results of the work of that conference were published as the sixth edition of the *International Classification of Diseases, Injuries, and Causes of Death* (ICD–6; WHO, 1949). This meeting was the beginning of a new era in international disease classification. In addition to approving a comprehensive taxonomy of both mortality and morbidity, that is, both death and disease, it promoted international cooperation in gathering health statistics worldwide. Over the 4 decades from 1949 to 1992, four subsequent revisions of the ICD were developed. An important development in terms of diagnosis in mental health began in 1978, when the WHO entered into a collaborative project with the U.S. Alcohol, Drug Abuse, and Mental Health Administration with the goal of improving the process of diagnosis in the area of mental health (WHO, 1993). The ICD–10, which included the advances made in the diagnosis of mental health disorders, was approved for use by the World Health Assembly in 1992, and the plan is to publish the 11th edition (ICD–11) in 2017.

The ICD today constitutes the standard in the world for categorizing and reporting diseases, health-related conditions, and external causes of disease and injury. It should be noted that the ninth edition (ICD–9) was adopted in 1979, and although the ICD–10 was adopted by most of the world after 1992, the ICD–9 continued to be used in the United States until October 1, 2015. That means that as of October 1, 2015, all entities covered by the Health Insurance Portability and Accountability Act of 1996 (HIPAA), including Medicare and Medicaid providers, are required to use the Clinical Modification of the ICD–10 (ICD–10–CM; National Center for Health Statistics, 2015) as their primary diagnostic system for purposes of reporting diseases and submitting claims for reimbursement by insurance companies. Most private insurers are likely to switch entirely to the ICD–10–CM system, which has substantial changes from the ICD–9. This means that it is likely that virtually every psychologist will be required to use the ICD–10–CM diagnostic system for billing and communication purposes, either directly or through translation programs from the *Diagnostic and Statistical Manual of Mental Disorders* (fifth ed.; *DSM–5*; American Psychiatric Association, 2013).

The ICD–10–CM

The ICD as published by the WHO is primarily a document intended to assist in compiling health-related data and providing a basis for research. Recognizing that the use in clinical contexts can require additional specificity, the WHO has authorized each country to publish its own adaptation of the ICD that meets the needs of clinicians in that country. The U.S. government, through the Centers for Medicare and Medicaid Services (CMS) (2015a, b), and the National Center for Health Statistics, both within the U.S. Department of Health and Human Services (DHHS), publishes the ICD–10–CM to meet that need. The purpose of this modification of the ICD is to provide a basis for classifying all visits to any health care facility or practitioner. The ICD–10–CM is the classification system that is discussed in this text. This document is available in PDF format free of charge from the U.S. government's Centers for Disease Control and Prevention at http://www.cdc.gov/nchs/icd/icd10cm.htm. Click on the FY2016 release, then the PDF Format, then in the resulting download, the Tabular PDF.

In addition to the ICD–10–CM, we refer to the *ICD–10 Classification of Mental and Behavioural Disorders: Clinical Descriptions and Diagnostic Guidelines* (*Blue Book*; WHO, 1993), the international document that provides a description of the main clinical features of all of the diagnoses in Chapter 5 of the ICD–10. The *Blue Book* is available free of charge from the WHO at the following website: http://www.who.int/classifications/icd/en/bluebook.pdf. In general, the ICD is designed for flexible use by clinicians, who are assumed to have expertise in mental health assessment, but the *Blue Book* can also be of use to clinicians in deciding between various diagnoses. We recommend that you download these two documents now and use them as you read this text.

The Basics of the ICD

The ICD model is referred to as a *variable-axis classification system*, which means that a certain number of categories provide a general structure to the system. One general category, for example, reflected in the middle chapters of the ICD–10–CM (Chapters 6–14), includes diseases having to do with specific anatomical locations, such as diseases of the eye or of the digestive system. Another general category is even more multifaceted, including external causes, such as injuries; constitutional diseases, such as cancer; developmental disorders, such as congenital problems; and epidemic diseases. Of most relevance to our discussion is Chapter 5, "Mental, Behavioral, and Neurodevelopmental Disorders," which includes the 11 subcategories contained in Exhibit 1.1.

The ICD–10–CM is composed of three volumes. Volume 1 is a listing of all diagnoses within the categories just described. It consists of 21 chapters that cover the major illnesses and causes of diseases within the ICD system. Volume 2 is an instruction manual, from which much of the current information is extracted, and Volume 3 is an alphabetical listing of all diagnoses to assist the professional in finding the appropriate diagnosis. That is, if you have the description of the diagnosis in mind and need to know the code (the combination of letters and numbers), use Volume 3 to find the correct code. For example, if you knew that the diagnosis was some form of anxiety, rather than looking for anxiety disorders within Chapter 5 of Volume 1, you could look for anxiety in the alphabetical listing of diseases in Volume 3 (found on p. 96). Because the online or downloadable form of Volume 1 has easy-to-use links (e.g.,

---

EXHIBIT 1.1

Categories of Mental, Behavioral, and Neurodevelopmental Disorders

1. Mental disorders due to known physiological conditions (F01–F09)
2. Mental and behavioral disorders due to psychoactive substance use (F10–F19)
3. Schizophrenia, schizotypal, delusional, and other non-mood psychotic disorders (F20–F29)
4. Mood [affective] disorders (F30–F39)
5. Anxiety, dissociative, stress-related, somatoform and other nonpsychotic mental disorders (F40–F48)
6. Behavioral syndromes associated with physiological disturbances and physical factors (F50–F59)
7. Disorders of adult personality and behavior (F60–F69)
8. Intellectual disabilities (F70–F79)
9. Pervasive and specific developmental disorders (F80–F89)
10. Behavioral and emotional disorders with onset usually occurring in childhood and adolescence (F90–F98)
11. Unspecified mental disorder (F99)

---

clicks on the blue print in the Table of Contents on p. 1 of Volume 1 to get to Chapter 5, then click on the blue print that immediately appears for Anxiety, dissociative, stress-related, somatoform and other nonpsychotic mental disorders to get to that section), in terms of ease of access, Volume 3 has few advantages for the mental health professional over Volume 1. However, Volume 3 lists various forms of the disorder that may be found elsewhere in Chapter 5, such as Separation anxiety of childhood (F93.0),[1] or symptoms that may be relevant that are not in Chapter 5, such as Depression: functional activity (R68.89). On the other hand, the listing of disorders under a general heading can include nonmental health disorders, which can be confusing. For example, under Depression (p. 360 in Volume 3) is also listed such physical disorders as bone marrow depression (D75.89) or chest wall depression (M95.4). For a well-trained mental health professional, it will be obvious those are medical disorders, not mental health disorders. Volume 3 has four sections contained in Exhibit 1.2. The section most relevant to psychology is the Index of Diseases and Injury.

---

[1]In this text, diagnostic terms in the ICD–10–CM are listed with the title of the diagnosis, with the first word capitalized, followed by the alphanumeric code: for example, Major depressive disorder, single episode, mild (F32.0). Such an alphanumeric code following a diagnostic label with the first word capitalized is taken directly from the coding of the ICD–10–CM.

EXHIBIT 1.2

Sections of ICD, Volume 3

Index of External Causes of Injury
Table of Neoplasms
Table of Drugs and Chemicals
Index of Diseases and Injury

The ICD–10–CM Coding System

The ICD–10–CM diagnosis codes consist of a series of letters and numbers, with a range from A00.00 to Z99.99. The first character is always a letter and designates the general category of the disorder. This constitutes a change from the ICD–9 (and differs from the DSM system) that used only numeric codes, hence the increasing divergence between the two systems.

The ICD–10–CM coding system, in comparison with the ICD–9, allows for an increase in the number of diagnoses listed (i.e., all diagnoses, psychiatric and general medical and surgical diagnoses) from somewhat more than 14,000 to slightly more than 69,000. In the portion of the ICD having to do with psychological disorders, the number of three-character diagnoses increased from 30 in the ICD–9 to 100 in the ICD–10, although some areas have fewer codes. For example, mood-related disorders has 78 full codes (four- to five-character codes) in the ICD–9–CM and 71 codes in the ICD–10–CM. On the other hand, the ICD–9–CM has one code for Other, whereas the ICD–10–CM has five subcategories, with each subcategory having from two to five subcategories under it. Thus, the general expansion enables greater specificity and more information in each diagnostic code, which enables improvements in tracking public health, making clinical decisions, and providing health care to patients. Many clinicians, however, will use only a small number of codes that are relevant to their specific practices.

In the ICD–10–CM coding system, Chapter 1, "Certain Infectious and Parasitic Diseases," has codes that begin with either the letter *A* or the letter *B*; Chapter 2, "Neoplasms" (cancers), has codes that begin with the letter *C*, and so on. All diagnoses that fall within Chapter 5, "Mental, Behavioral, and Neurodevelopmental Disorders," begin with the letter *F*. This chapter (Codes F01–F99; pp. 193–234 in the document you have downloaded from the WHO website) is most relevant to the issues discussed in this book. The other diagnostic categories with relevance to mental health symptoms begin with the letter *R*, (R40–R49),

T (T74–T79), and *Z* (Z02–Z04) and are contained in Chapter 18, pages 948–953; Chapter 19, pages 1356–1360; and Chapter 21, pages 1538–1539, respectively.

The next two characters in the ICD code, the first of which is always numeric, are the specific diagnoses within the general category. The ICD–10–CM attempts to group conditions together that have a common theme, making it easy to find diagnoses. For example, mood disorders have one of the codes F30–F39: Manic episode (F30), Bipolar disorder (F31), Major depressive disorder (F32), and so on. Thus, the fundamental coding system of the ICD–10–CM includes three characters and a letter designating the general category, followed by two characters, the first of which is numeric and the second of which is either numeric or alphabetic, designating the specific diagnosis. In the case of mental health disorders (see Chapter 5 of ICD–10) or symptoms (see Chapter 18 of ICD–10), however, both of the next two characters are numeric. Some of the diagnostic codes are for classes of disorders, whereas some are for single conditions, which usually reflect diseases that occur frequently, are severe, or have specific interventions associated with them.

General diagnoses can have subcategories, which are designated by a series of characters that follow a decimal point and which in the mental health area, Chapters 5 and 18 of the ICD–10–CM are all numeric. Subcategories can designate either a specific type of a disorder or the severity of the disorder. Thus, Bipolar disorder, current episode manic without psychotic features is coded F31.1; Bipolar disorder, current episode manic severe with psychotic features is F31.2; and so on. The fourth character .8 is generally used for "other" conditions belonging to the three-character category. Thus, F31.8 is Other bipolar disorders. The fourth character .9 is the "unspecified" designation; for example, F31.9 is Bipolar disorders, unspecified. In some cases, the subcategory is further categorized, allowing for a second, third, or fourth number following the decimal, reflecting greater differentiation between subcategories. In this example, if the symptoms of the bipolar disorder without psychotic features are mild, the coding is F30.11; if moderate, F30.12; and if severe, F30.13. Likewise, the code F40.2 is Specific (isolated) phobias. The subcategory Animal type phobias is coded F40.21 and subcategories of that code are 40.210, Arachnophobia (fear of spiders), and 40.218, Other animal type phobias.

If a particular diagnosis does not have a second number following the decimal, it is recommended that an *x* be placed in that location when submitting a diagnosis, such as Bipolar disorder, current episode manic severe with psychotic features (F31.2x). On the other hand, if a diagnosis has two or more numbers following the decimal, the entire code must be used. For example, posttraumatic stress disorder (PTSD) has three specific manifestations, PTSD unspecified (F43.10), PTSD acute (F43.11), and PTSD chronic (F43.12). One of those codes must be used. A coding of F43.1 alone will not be considered a valid coding.

If more than one diagnostic code is appropriate, the code listed first is considered the primary or principal diagnosis for that particular *patient encounter*, which is the term used in the ICD for all patient contacts, whether inpatient or outpatient and whether the purpose is assessment or treatment. If other diagnoses are present, but those were not considered or were not the primary focus during a particular encounter, they should be listed as secondary diagnostic codes.

Additional ICD–10–CM Coding Designations

In addition to the general rubric, that is, the three-, four-, or five-character code and title of the diagnosis, a few additional designations help clarify the diagnostic category and distinguish it from alternative diagnoses. In some diagnoses the term *includes* or *excludes* is used. Thus, under F30, the diagnosis *Manic episode* clarifies that it includes *bipolar disorder, single manic episode* and *mixed affective episode* but excludes *Bipolar disorder (F31.—)*,[2] *Major depressive disorder, single episode (F32.—)*, and *Major depressive disorder, recurrent (F33.—)*. In the case of the exclusion category, the diagnosis being excluded is listed in some other category and the coding of the alternative diagnoses is provided, with the dash replacing the specific subcategory that should also be included. In this example, *Bipolar disorder (F31.—)* is considered a separate diagnostic category, not part of the category, *F30, Manic episode*. If the presentation in a particular encounter is manic, but part of a varying presentation of nonpsychotic mania and depression, the appropriate diagnostic category would be *F31.1x, Bipolar disorder, current episode manic without psychotic features*, with the x being replaced by the number appropriately reflecting the severity of the presentation (F31.10 = unspecified severity, F31.11 = mild severity, F31.12 = moderate severity, and F31.13 = severe).

The first of two types of exclusion categories is *Excludes1*, which means that the code to be excluded should never be listed as a diagnosis with the primary diagnosis, because the two diagnoses cannot occur together. *Excludes2* means that the excluded code is not the same as or part of the diagnosis with which it is listed, but a person can have both

---

[2]A dash indicates that a number of subcategories (subtypes) are possible within the code.

conditions, so both codes could be listed as diagnoses. For example, under *F32, Major depressive disorder, single episode,* is *Excludes1: Bipolar disorder (F31.—),* meaning that a person cannot be given both the diagnosis *Major depressive disorder (F32)* and *Bipolar disorder (F31.—).* Also under F32 is *Excludes2: Adjustment disorder (F43.2),* meaning that F43.2 is a different diagnosis from F32 but that a patient could be given both diagnoses because they are different but not mutually exclusive.

Brackets are used to designate synonyms or alternative wording, as in *Mood [affective] disorders.* Parentheses are used to indicate supplemental, but nonessential, modifiers, such as in *Other specified anxiety disorders, Anxiety depression (mild or not persistent)* or to reflect the coding for a diagnosis that is an exclusion, such as indicated in the preceding paragraph.

When a condition has an underlying etiology (cause), with multiple manifestations (presentations), the ICD uses the designation "use additional code," with the etiology (underlying cause) code to indicate that the specific manifestation of that underlying cause should also be listed as a diagnosis. For example, in the category F84, *Pervasive developmental disorders,* it states: "Use additional code to identify any associated medical condition and intellectual disabilities." This means that this category could be the result of or be associated with a medical condition, which should also be listed, and could have intellectual implications, which should also be listed, if appropriate. So, for example, a child could have a developmental disorder as a result of a *Bacterial meningitis* (coded G00, found in Chapter 6, ICD–10–CM), which could be coded, if known, and could have effects on intellectual functioning, such as a *Moderate intellectual disability (F71).*

The ICD uses the term *code first* with the manifestation code to indicate that the underlying cause of the disorder should be listed as the first diagnosis. Usually in this instance, the term *in other diseases classified elsewhere* is used to indicate that this is one manifestation of another, more basic, disease entity. For example, under F01, *Vascular dementia,* it states, "Code first the underlying physiological condition or sequelae of cerebrovascular disease," meaning that the underlying cardiovascular disorder that causes the vascular dementia should be listed as the primary diagnosis, such as *Systolic (congestive) heart failure (I50.2),* as one example. Obviously, a medical diagnosis would be provided by a physician, not a psychologist.

The term *code also* is used to indicate that another diagnostic code should typically be used to describe fully the disorder being considered, although this term does not indicate which code should be the primary diagnosis. This is to be determined by the clinician, considering all of the data available from the assessment. Likewise, if more than one diagnostic code can be established with equal support from the clinical data, either of the codes can be listed as primary. For example, *Pain disorder with related psychological factors (F45.42)* directs the clinician to code also *associated acute or chronic pain (G89.—)*, providing the code of the disorder that should also be listed.

It should be noted that a distinction is made in the ICD–10–CM between *Not otherwise specified (NOS)*, on the one hand, a diagnosis without specific qualifications that does not meet all of the requirements of another diagnosis, and, on the other hand, *Not elsewhere classified (NEC)*, meaning that certain types of the diagnosis may occur elsewhere. The specification NOS in the ICD–10–CM has the same meaning as NOS in the previous versions of the *DSM* system classifications through the fourth edition, text revision, of the *DSM (DSM–IV*; American Psychiatric Association, 2000), but NOS was eliminated from the *DSM–5*. In the current *DSM*, the designation NEC is used when a specific code is not available for the condition or in other words, for understudied conditions (Brown, Keel, & Striegel, 2012). In the ICD–10–CM, the designation *Not elsewhere classified* is used in Chapter 5 only in the general exclusion category at the very beginning of the chapter, where it refers to sets of signs and symptoms that do not have a specific diagnosis, that is, it refers to Chapter 18, with codes of R00–R99. On the other hand, the phrase *classified elsewhere* does occur frequently in Chapter 5 and refers to a diagnosis that is a result of some other condition, and the other condition should also be listed, often as the primary diagnosis. For example, *Dementia in other diseases classified elsewhere (F02)* includes dementia as a result of other conditions, such as Alzheimer's disease (G30.—). In this example, when a diagnosis of dementia is given and is the result of another condition, such as *Alzheimer's disease*, the underlying physiological condition should be listed as the primary diagnosis and dementia should be listed as a secondary diagnosis. However, it is also important to note that the clinician should use as many diagnostic codes as necessary to present an accurate picture of the individual's level of functioning. Generally, which diagnoses are given precedence is dependent on which will be most useful or helpful, given the purpose of the assessment or which is most predominant in a given encounter.

General Considerations in Diagnosing

Whenever possible, specific diagnostic codes should be used. However, sometimes, the information available is insufficient to establish a specific diagnosis. In that case, two possible types of codes can be used. In the case when a number of signs (what is observed by the clinician, the objective data) and symptoms (what is reported by the patient, the subjective data) are present but insufficient in number or in specificity to establish a definitive diagnosis, codes with the terms *unspecified* or *NOS* can be used, as in Major depressive disorder, single episode, unspecified (F32.9). This is used when some of the signs and symptoms of a major depressive disorder are present but not sufficient in number to establish a more specific diagnosis of Major depressive disorder (F32.x). Sometimes, specific signs and symptoms are present, but without a sufficient configuration of symptoms to warrant even an unspecified diagnosis. Chapter 18 of the ICD–10–CM provides a listing of such signs and symptoms with associated codes. For example, without sufficient indication of a Sleeping disorder (F51.xx), the sole symptoms of Somnolence (drowsiness) has a code of R40.0. Some additional useful examples of such categories used by psychologists are Age-related cognitive decline (R41.81), Auditory hallucinations (R44.0), Unhappiness (R45.2; not meeting all of the requirements for Depression), Hostility (R45.5), Violent behavior (R45.6), and Suspiciousness and marked evasiveness (R46.5). Thus, if the psychologist observes or is aware of a series of specific behaviors or emotional states that are relevant but are not sufficient for a specific diagnosis, Chapter 18 (and in particular, R40–R46, Symptoms and signs involving cognition, perception, emotional state, and behavior) should be consulted for useful coding. However, if a definitive diagnosis has been established, that diagnosis should be used as the primary diagnosis.

We emphasize that for all diagnoses, whether specific, unspecified, or based on one sign or symptoms, the specific problems or complaints observed during an encounter and a sufficient basis in observed or reported facts should be present and documentation provided to assign any diagnostic code to a patient's condition. However, what is one to do when there are not yet sufficient data to provide a definitive diagnosis but the data do suggest some hypotheses of what an appropriate diagnosis might be? Often, such terms as *rule out* or *suspected* or *probable* would be used. In the ICD system, the correct thing to do is to use the code (even a definitive diagnosis) that is suspected as if it were already established, with documentation of a specific plan for continuing the assessment to gather more information.

In an encounter without a specific diagnosis providing the reason for that encounter, Chapter 21, "Factors Influencing Health Status and Contact With Health Services," provides codes appropriate to such situations (all of these diagnoses have codes beginning with the letter Z). Relevant to work a psychologist might do, there are codes for premarital counseling (Z02.89: Encounter for other administrative examinations), initial assessments following a rape to determine whether a diagnosis is appropriate (Z04.4x: Encounter for examination and observation following alleged rape), initial forensic assessments without findings of a psychological disorder (Z04.6: Encounter for general psychiatric examination, requested by authority, or Z04.8: Encounter for examination and observation for other specified reasons) or a general screening (Z13.9: Encounter for general screening, unspecified).

Why the ICD?

Why does this book use the ICD–10–CM as its diagnostic manual? Don't most American psychologists use the *DSM–5*? The answer to the second question is, or in the past has been, yes. The first question has a number of answers. First, the ICD–10–CM is the classification system in mental health that is the official diagnostic system for mental and behavioral disorders in the United States, including those codes used by Medicare and required by HIPAA. In addition to its use by the U.S. government, it is the classification system used by and required by most private insurance companies.

Most psychologists would likely say that the official diagnostic system in the United States is the *DSM–5*. And, in fact, when the *DSM–IV* was in effect, it corresponded virtually identically with the ICD–9–CM classification codes (the numbers used to identify the diagnosis). So, when a practitioner diagnosed someone using a DSM–IV diagnosis and submitted the corresponding code to the insurance company, the insurance company simply read it as an ICD–9–CM code—no problem. However, the move to the ICD–10–CM and the *DSM–5* has led to some increased divergence between the two coding systems; acknowledging this divergence, the *DSM–5* has included ICD–9–CM and ICD–10–CM codes with the *DSM–5* codes. When the international community moves to the ICD–11, which is anticipated to begin in 2017, there is likely to be even more divergence; because one of the goals of the ICD–11 is to make the classifications of even more practical use to the clinician, additional changes will probably be needed to the current systems. Therefore, it will become increasingly incumbent on psychologists practicing in the United States who submit bills to insurance companies to become acquainted with and use the ICD coding system.

Second, the ICD is the classification system used in the rest of the world. Ninety-five percent of physicians, nurses, and psychologists in the world use the ICD system (Reed, 2013). In fact, all of the member countries of the WHO (including the United States and Canada) are required by international treaty to collect health data and report those data to the WHO using the ICD classification system. So, both to be in compliance with international treaties and to operate consistent with the rest of the world, it will become increasingly important for psychologists in the United States to use the ICD framework.

Third, by using the ICD system, North American health practitioners will be contributing to a consistent and systematic way of tracking and treating health-related dysfunctions. Thus, they will contribute to the attainment of maximal health throughout the world.

Fourth, the reader has learned in this chapter that the ICD system is quite user friendly for both experienced and novice users. And that it is the standard used by the federal government and most insurance companies, as well as the rest of the world. So, becoming versed in the ICD system makes sense. Nevertheless, as with any skill, to become competent in the implementation of this classification system in your clinical work, you will need to implement your knowledge through supervised practice.

Psychological Assessment
The Foundation for Diagnosis

2

In this chapter, we focus on the myriad challenges to being objective and accurate in our assessment of patients. We begin by discussing views of abnormality and defining and describing the process of diagnosis. We then explore the issues involved in the process of assessment, in particular, common cognitive errors.

What Is Abnormal?

The world is increasingly diverse, yet connected. With increased awareness of diversity, people have become cognizant of the risks associated with human prejudice (Collins & Clément, 2012; Gordijn, Finchilescu, Brix, Wijnants, & Koomen, 2008; Hogg & Williams, 2000; Murphy, Richeson, Shelton, Reinschmidt, & Bergsieker, 2013; Richeson & Shelton, 2007;

http://dx.doi.org/10.1037/14778-003
A Student's Guide to Assessment and Diagnosis Using the ICD–10–CM: Psychological and Behavioral Conditions, by J. Schaffer and E. Rodolfa

EXHIBIT 2.1

Factors Influencing Views of Abnormality

Frequency of behavior
Subjective distress
Deviation from societal norms
Risk
Interference with social functioning

Tajfel & Turner, 1986). With this awareness of, and increasing acceptance of, human diversity (Teixeira & Halpin, 2013), what value does it have for us as professionals and for society to regard some individuals, whose behavior is diverse in particular ways, as possessing a psychological problem, otherwise referred to as a "mental health diagnosis"?

How do we know or decide that a particular individual should appropriately be viewed as having a psychological condition? How do we set aside particular types of diverse behaviors and fit them into a different category, one that we categorize as problematic? What are the criteria for making such a decision, one that can have dramatic effects on the recipient of this label? We discuss some of these criteria in the following subsections. Exhibit 2.1 provides an overview of the criteria we can rely on to help us decide whether a behavior is problematic in some way.

FREQUENCY

Certainly, the frequency of the behavior is one consideration (Oyebode, 2008). If a behavior is statistically unusual, it is more likely to be considered abnormal. However, behaviors can occur infrequently for a variety of reasons. People behave in certain ways in response to environmental stimuli or demands. If an environmental event is unusual, say, being held up on the street at gunpoint, which for most people is a rare occurrence, thankfully, our response to such an event is likely to be unusual (e.g., passive compliance or, at the other end of the spectrum, verbal or behavioral aggression), but whatever the response, it might be very appropriate and adaptive, depending on the situation and the outcome.

Likewise, the behavior by a person from a different culture might be unusual in a North American culture but common in that culture. Would such unusual behavior be worthy of a psychological diagnosis? Almost certainly not, but for the presence of considerable cultural insensitivity (Alarcón, 2009). Or if a behavior is unusual but appropriate given the context or circumstances (e.g., locking oneself in a room—in the context of an abusive family member), that almost certainly would not be considered psychologically abnormal. In fact, it might be the most psychologically adaptive response to a challenging situation.

Another way of thinking about the frequency issue, in addition to frequency of a behavior, for a group of people or a culture is the typicality of the behavior for the individual. If a behavior constitutes an abnormal one for the individual—that is, it is unusual for that person, given that person's history of cognitions, behaviors, and emotions—such a behavior is more likely to be considered appropriate for a psychological diagnosis. But, again, if the circumstances are new or uncommon, the unusual behavior may be adaptive. In an otherwise self-confident, assertive person, passivity and compliance in the face of a gun may be normal and adaptive and normally assertive behavior might be deadly. So, if frequency by itself is an insufficient criterion, what else is required?

SUBJECTIVE DISTRESS

Yet another consideration in whether a behavior is abnormal is the subjective distress of the individual. *Subjective distress* is a term used to describe emotions that interfere with a patient's—or more broadly, a person's—ability to function. As everyone manifests subjective distress differently, it is important to understand the contributing factors to and implications of subjective distress on an individual's life.

For instance, if a person is upset by, or uncomfortable with, the emotions or cognitions she or he experiences when engaging in a particular behavior, then that behavior is more likely to be thought of as abnormal. Certainly, subjective distress is one important element of abnormality. In fact, if the level of subjective distress is high enough and interferes with daily functioning, some kind of psychological abnormality is highly likely. However, as a counterexample, both of us have lost parents in the past few years, which resulted in very upsetting, but perfectly normal and adaptive, emotions. So, although distressing emotions may be a necessary element of abnormality, they are not sufficient.

DEVIATION FROM SOCIETAL NORMS

Likewise, deviation from societal norms is a factor to take into account. This is not quite the same as frequency, because a behavior could be infrequent but still not violate social norms. At the same time, one must remember that abnormal behavior is not necessarily mental illness. Criminal behavior is abnormal and violates social norms but in and of itself is not a mental illness. Likewise, rebelliousness in an adolescent, although often disturbing to those around him or her, is not by itself an indication of a mental illness. Similarly, rebelliousness against an oppressive societal norm, for example, defiance in the face of the violent racism often expressed during the era of slavery in 19th century America, is not a mental illness.

RISK

Another consideration is whether the behavior places the physical or psychological well-being of someone at risk. For instance, deep feelings of depression sap one's motivation to do much of anything and, therefore, may even place one's life at risk because one may draw the conclusion that continuing to live is not worth the effort. Or, hallucinations, especially if they involve violent images, might influence people to harm others and, in turn, create a risk to people in proximity to the person experiencing the hallucinations. On the other hand, the rebelliousness against slavery that often occurred (see Northup, 1855) most definitely resulted in risk to the rebellious slave but was by no means the result of a mental illness. In fact, from today's perspective of resilience (Reich, Zautra, & Hall, 2010), it likely would be considered a strength.

INTERFERENCE WITH SOCIAL FUNCTIONING

Yet another factor that is considered an important element of abnormality is whether the behavior, cognition, or emotion in some way interferes with the individual's ability to function adequately in his or her social context (e.g., Aetna, 2015; Beidel, Frueh, & Hersen, 2014; Centers for Medicare and Medicaid Services, 2015b). A number of terms or concepts in that sentence require greater specificity to provide clarity and avoid confusion. How much of an impediment to "normal" functioning does the behavior have to cause? How uncharacteristic does the behavior have to be for it to be considered abnormal? If an abnormality is dependent on the social context, is the concept of abnormal totally dependent on social norms and expectations, or are aspects of behavior considered abnormal regardless of context?

Given the complexity of human behavior and human social systems, these questions do not have definitive answers. Many variables influence when a behavior is considered a mental disorder. To come to a conclusion regarding a specific individual, which is one of the first and most important tasks of the psychologist, one needs a starting point, a foundation from which to make judgments. The Clinical Modification of the *International Statistical Classification of Diseases and Related Health Problems* (ICD–10–CM; National Center for Health Statistics, 2015) provides such a foundation for understanding unusual behaviors by providing a standardized, internationally accepted definition of what types of unusual behaviors fall into a category we refer to as "mental illness."

What Is a Diagnosis?

What value does diagnosis have, and does diagnosis carry any disadvantages? First, one should consider the question, What is a diagnosis? In medical terms, a *diagnosis* is a cluster of symptoms that typically occur together in the presence of some underlying anatomical, physiological, or biochemical abnormality. The diagnosis is used to describe and explain the problems the patient presents. Thus, for example, a person with blocked (occluded) coronary arteries will have symptoms such as pain or pressure in the chest (angina) or other parts of the upper body, shortness of breath, nausea, and profuse sweating (diaphoresis). A single term, the diagnosis, is used to convey information about that constellation of symptoms, all of which have the same underlying cause. In medicine, the diagnosis is necessary for treatment, as it points the way to the appropriate intervention strategy.

How does considering the use of diagnosis by physicians relate to the practice of psychology? Many or most psychological abnormalities do not fit all of the typical requirements of a medical diagnosis. Although they have been considered at least in part related to the nervous system since the fifth century B.C.E. (Alcmaeon, a Greek medical scientist and philosopher, discussed them in such terms; Millon, 1969), the specific anatomical, physiological, and biochemical dysfunctions that underlie psychological disorders have not yet been unequivocally identified. Thus, although a cardiologist may have a good idea of what is going on physically when a person presents with angina, a psychologist does not know precisely what is happening anatomically or physiologically when a person presents as depressed; what psychologists have at this point are hypotheses.

Psychologists must also consider that although a very large number of symptoms can be present in any particular disorder, a given individual may present with only a small number of them. For the diagnosis major depressive disorder (MDD), the *Diagnostic and Statistical Manual of Mental Disorders* (fifth ed.; *DSM–5*; American Psychiatric Association, 2013) lists nine symptoms. To obtain the diagnosis of MDD, one has to present with five or more of those nine symptoms, with one of the five symptoms being either depressed mood or loss of interest or pleasure. That means that, taking five symptoms at a time, as many as 72 different combinations of symptoms could result in the diagnosis of MDD, whereas in the fourth edition of the *DSM* (American Psychiatric Association, 2000), it was 126 combinations. Thus, currently, a person could be diagnosed with MDD up to 72 different ways, quite different from an occlusion in a coronary artery that results in chronic chest pain (e.g., chronic ischemic heart disease; coded in ICD–10–CM as I25), which itself is a much more nonspecific diagnosis than many cardiac diagnoses (e.g., see ST elevation myocardial infarction of the anterior wall, I21.0). The ICD–10–CM does not have quite the same problem, because it does not adopt the same menu approach (choosing x number of symptoms from a list of y number of symptoms). However, any diagnostic classification system will have limits in the amount of information the diagnostic label itself can convey.

Thus, a psychological diagnosis is a summary statement or a conceptual inference (i.e., a hypothetical construct)—something useful but not observable with the five human senses (Cronbach & Meehl, 1955)—for a cluster of symptoms that provides a mental health professional an understanding of the relevant problems experienced by the patient. And, most notably, it means that the diagnostic category by itself has much more limited value for us as psychologists because of the minimal information the diagnostic label provides us about who this individual we are working with is and what we need to understand to be helpful. Much more on that important issue below.

Purposes of Diagnosis

Psychological diagnosis has a number of very concrete and positive purposes, as listed in Exhibit 2.2. Certainly, the first and foremost purpose of diagnosis must be an understanding of the patient. By engaging in the diagnostic process, psychologists gather important information about the individuals with whom they work professionally. Understanding the types of symptoms that combine to make a diagnostic category helps us as psychologists think about the types of problems that a given individual may be experiencing. Such understandings help us formulate questions about the person's experience that might not otherwise occur to us but that help us understand the person better and ultimately lead to a more appropriate disposition.

On a very practical level, diagnosis is necessary for insurance reimbursement and is one reason many clinicians attach diagnostic labels to their patients. Insurance companies determine the criteria for reimburse-

EXHIBIT 2.2

Purposes of Diagnosis

Understanding the patient
Communication through common language
Inform the treatment process
Insight into possible causes of disorders

ment and have stipulated that a service must be "medically necessary" to be eligible for reimbursement. The U.S. federal government's definition of *medically necessary* is brief and simple: "Services or supplies that are needed to diagnose or treat your medical condition and that meet accepted standards of medical practice" (Medicare, 2013). As an additional example, Anthem Blue Cross, the trade name of Blue Cross in California, adds some more specific requirements:

> "Medical Necessity" shall mean health care services that a medical practitioner, exercising prudent clinical judgment, would provide to a Covered Individual for the purpose of preventing, evaluating, diagnosing or treating an illness, injury, disease or its symptoms, and that are
>
> (a) in accordance with generally accepted standards of medical practice;
> (b) clinically appropriate . . .; and
> (c) not primarily for the convenience of the Covered Individual, physician, or other health care provider;
> (d) and not more costly than an alternative service. . . .
>
> For these purposes, "generally accepted standards of medical practice" means standards that are based on credible scientific evidence published in peer-reviewed medical literature generally recognized by the relevant medical community . . . and the views of medical practitioners practicing in relevant clinical areas and any other relevant factors

An essential element of this language is that one cannot be careless or nonchalant about giving someone a diagnosis. Specific expectations about the evidence underlie a diagnosis and rules about how one goes about the process of diagnosing. In addition to doing potential harm to the patient, not following those rules can mean, at best, that a claim submitted for insurance reimbursement will be rejected and, at worst, that the clinician can be accused of fraudulent billing.

The primary value of diagnosis in a clinical setting is its ability to communicate a considerable amount of information in a brief manner. Communicating to another professional the diagnosis of an individual provides a great deal of information about the person's experiences and presentation, without having to list all of the observed behaviors (Trull, 2005). Such shorthand communication not only enables another professional to have some understanding of the patient but also to have a certain level of empathy for the individual's experience. In turn, it can provide patients some understanding of why they have the kinds of experiences they have and, thereby, allows them to be less critical or judgmental and more accepting of themselves.

A related purpose of diagnosis is to have a common language and consistent means of talking about specific behaviors, cognitions, and emotions, with some limitations discussed below. Not only does diagnosis allow clinicians to communicate information to each other, but it also ensures that professions are generally talking about the same types of events when using specific terminology. It is often the case in everyday conversation that people use words with slightly different nuances, a fact that a clinician ignores with some risk to therapeutic effectiveness. However, diagnostic systems such as the ICD–10–CM enable psychologists to use well-defined terms in the same way, such that the probability of misunderstanding is diminished. In addition, the ICD–10–CM enables research into certain types of problems to develop more effective treatments for problems. In 1967, Gordon Paul asked the question regarding psychotherapy that has become the prototypic question of researchers and clinicians alike: "What treatment, by whom, is most effective for this individual with that specific problem, and under which set of circumstances?" (p. 111). Having an accurate diagnosis is an essential first step in answering that question. Having at least a partial answer is essential for being able to provide effective psychological service or intervention.

The single most important purpose of diagnosis for us as psychologists is to inform the treatment process. In short, one cannot know what treatment is appropriate without knowing the nature of the problem being treated. Thus, the process of reaching a diagnosis helps in identifying and clarifying the nature of the problem, including its severity, complexity, and impact on daily functioning, and assists the clinician in setting therapeutic goals as a function of the problems presented.

Having stated all of that, we also believe that the value a diagnosis has for psychological treatment, which focuses on the individual and his or her experience and specific behaviors, can be somewhat limited because the presence of a diagnosis per se is inadequate to distinguish one person from another, that is, one person with major depression from another, given all of the ways a person can end up with that diagnosis. In the absence of specific insights into the behaviors of a particular individual, the contribution of diagnosis to our work as psychologists can at times be minimal. That is, the most central part of diagnosis for psychologists is the assessment process and the interplay between diagnosis and data collection that accompany the development of a diagnosis. We discuss this process at greater length below.

Last, although the science of causality in human behavior is still young, diagnostic categories can give us some insight into possible causes of the presenting symptoms and can raise questions in our minds about which avenues to pursue in a search for causality. This is true not only for the clinician working with a specific client but also for the researcher searching for the underlying causes of all psychological diagnoses.

However, the degree to which the diagnosis per se is helpful to psychologists is dependent in part on the setting and the nature of the diagnosis. In many settings, such as college counseling centers and small, private practices, the diagnostic category itself may provide little additional information, beyond the understanding of the person obtained through a process of adequate assessment, regarding the preferred treatment options, even though the diagnosis may be necessary for insurance reimbursement. In other settings—for example, multidisciplinary settings—the diagnosis may be central to the collaborative efforts across disciplines. Further, certain diagnoses, such as Paranoid schizophrenia (F20.0) or Bipolar disorder, current episode hypomanic (F31.0), do provide information that is central and critical to decisions about treatment.

Pitfalls of Diagnosis

The process of reaching a diagnosis includes a number of potential difficulties (see Exhibit 2.3). First, the empirical data regarding the reliability of diagnoses are not encouraging (Bhugra, Easter, Mallaris, & Gupta, 2011; Matuszak & Piasecki, 2012). For example, in one study, experienced psychiatrists, the vast majority of whom had used the diagnosis Schizoaffective disorder (F25.x in the ICD–10–CM), largely disagreed with each other regarding which symptoms are appropriate to the disorder, with more than half of the respondents disagreeing that it was a distinct diagnostic category, even though they had used it as a diagnosis (Rowe & Clark, 2008). Given the subjective nature of psychological diagnoses, and the large combinations of symptoms that can result in a single diagnosis, the consistency with which clinicians use the same diagnostic code is discouragingly low. How one clinician uses Major depressive disorder, recurrent, moderate (F33.1x) might be different from how another clinician understands it, such that miscommunication between the two professionals is still possible. As a result, the communicative power of diagnosis is not as high as desirable. One variable that explains some, although not all, of the variance in diagnosis is the presence of comorbidity; that is, it is often the case that more than one diagnosis

---

EXHIBIT 2.3

Pitfalls of Diagnosis

Reliability
Stigma
Labeling
Diagnostic categories are discrete
Arbitrary nature of diagnosis

may be present, resulting in complex interrelationships between symptoms in each individual (Borsboom, Cramer, Schmittmann, Epskamp, & Waldorp, 2011), which supports our contention above that the diagnostic label alone has limited value to us as psychologists.

Second, although stigma attached to psychiatric diagnoses is diminishing, it has not vanished (N. Evans, Gilpin, Holmes, Rafique, & Yates, 2010; Hayne, 2003; Lyons, Hopley, Horrocks, 2009). People with a psychiatric diagnosis are often viewed with caution or, even, paranoia (ironic, as paranoia is itself a symptom of a psychological disorder) and not treated the same way as "normals" (as if any of us would fall into that category!). Thus, individuals who have received a psychiatric diagnosis can sometimes be denied employment or housing or any other of many social necessities, even though doing so is against the Americans With Disabilities Act (2014). Attaching a diagnosis to an individual can create stigma that might follow that person for the rest of his or her life. Future disadvantages might outweigh the current advantages of having a diagnosis. Further, the patient cannot be expected to understand what either the current advantages or future disadvantages might be. It is incumbent on the clinician to be sensitive to such issues and, following the Hippocratic Oath (Hulkower, 2010) and Principle A of the *Ethical Principles of Psychologists and Code of Conduct* (American Psychological Association, 2010): First, do no harm.

A third related disadvantage of diagnosis is that applying a label to a person tends to make people view the person more as an entity than an individual. Each person has strengths and weaknesses. Certainly, the areas of weakness, inadequacy, or abnormality are major foci of any diagnostic enterprise. However, each person has her or his own pattern of weaknesses that come from specific environmental experiences. Without understanding something of those patterns and experiences, the label itself does not convey sufficient information about who the individual is and what his or her experiences are like. Equally as important, the label indicates nothing about the pattern of strengths—recognizing this is also necessary to understand the person, and without which a program of effective intervention is virtually impossible. Beyond such weaknesses of diagnosis, a diagnosis can blind the clinician to the complexity of the individual. Given the tendency to seek evidence that confirms one's impressions (see below), the diagnostic label might interfere with the psychologist's ability to gather additional information that will lead to a better understanding of the person, not to mention with the perceptions of nonprofessionals in the person's environment, and the characteristics implicit in the diagnosis may be self-fulfilling, as the person may come to expect such behaviors, cognitions, and emotions from himself or herself.

Fourth, diagnostic categories are by nature discrete. A person either fits into a category or not. One either is a graduate student or not. One either has a broken bone or not. Human behavior, cognitions, and emo-tions are, however, much more continuous than discrete. People can have varying degrees of anxiety or depression. As we discuss below, all people have varying degrees of irrational or inaccurate cognitions. Depending on the context, everyone has acted in a strange or unusual way at times. How does one decide at what point on a continuum one considers a person to have, for example, a Generalized anxiety disorder (F41.1)? How much anxiety is necessary? How disruptive or distressing must the anxiety be? Is the difference meaningful between a person who does not quite meet the criteria and a person who does but just barely?

Last is the arbitrary nature of the diagnostic enterprise in mental health. Most diagnoses are developed in a discussion of a committee of experts. Such discussions are not likely to be necessary in deciding whether a broken bone or a viral infection is a disease or not. Perhaps the stereotypical example of this problem was the inclusion of homo-sexuality as a disease in the first and second editions of the *DSM* (American Psychiatric Association, 1952, 1968) but its exclusion from the third (American Psychiatric Association, 1980) and subsequent editions of the *DSM*. The *Oxford Dictionary of American English* defines *disease* as "a disorder of structure or function in a human, animal, or plant, especially one that produces specific signs or symptoms or that affects a specific location and is not simply a direct result of physical injury" ("Disease," 2014). Wouldn't one expect such a condition to be an objective affliction that goes beyond what a committee of people can decide upon?

In addition to the advantages and disadvantages of attempting to diagnose an individual, the diagnostic process has some other pitfalls. When an individual first presents in a clinical context, the amount of information gathered is extensive and includes what the person says about his or her inner experiences, the way in which that informa-tion is presented (i.e., with or without emotion, level of certainty, the amount of force or energy inherent in the telling, etc.), the facts of the person's life as described by the patient, and the observations made by the professional, including developing hypotheses about the meaning or significance of the story being told and the other data being gath-ered. Sometimes the presence of one sign or symptom, referred to as a *pathognomonic sign*, is sufficient for a diagnosis. For example, if a person is clearly hallucinating, that is usually a strong indication that some abnormal process is occurring, although whether it is a result of a psychosis or drug use or some other cause might not be apparent. One must also recognize that in some circumstances (i.e., some cul-tures or religious contexts), what in a psychological context might be labeled a hallucination might be labeled a vision, a dream, or a trance and, therefore, not pathological (Benedict, 1934; Myers, 2011; see also Luhrmann, 2011; Luhrmann, Padmavati, Tharoor, & Osei, 2014).

In part because of the risk of misidentifying the experience, most often a diagnosis is arrived at by considering a broad range of data and the patterns observed in those data. Given the overwhelming amount of information being communicated, the clinician needs some framework for deciding both what is important and how the various elements of the data being presented fit together in a coherent whole that provides an understanding of the individual's experience. Thus, what is needed is a system that provides an objective classification of behaviors and experiences that assists the clinician in organizing, privileging, and interpreting the data available. The ICD–10–CM diagnostic system provides just such a framework agreed upon by international experts.

As we mentioned earlier, diagnoses in mental health are conceptual inferences. They are concepts or conclusions that the clinician comes to, on the basis of information gathered. One might even debate whether they exist "in the person," as Thomas Szasz (1961) argued in his classic book, in all but the most serious dysfunctions. They certainly do not present themselves like a broken bone that is projecting through the skin (a compound fracture) or, even, like a burst appendix that one cannot see by looking at the person (although what one would see by looking at a person with a burst appendix would certainly lead one to believe that something pretty serious is going on) but would be readily apparent through medical imaging. Rather, psychological diagnoses are based on a combination of data, including signs and symptoms, as well as a variety of other information (see Chapter 3, this volume, for a discussion about sources of psychological data). The clinician's task is to decide what kinds of data to collect and from whom or where; how to assess the data and follow up, as necessary, to clarify or add to the data collected; and then to conceptualize the data in a way that allows for reasonably reliable conclusions (meaning other professionals with the same data would likely come to the same conclusions) and valid conclusions (meaning they fit the individual in question) regarding the experiences and condition of the patient.

The Potential for Error

As might be obvious, this extremely complex process requires considerable knowledge, skill, and experience, as well as a conscious awareness of some of the factors that play an important role in whether the clinician's conclusions are reasonably reliable and valid, as the process of coming to a diagnosis can itself lead to some errors. Some of those factors that affect the accuracy of an assessment are listed in Exhibit 2.4.

EXHIBIT 2.4

The Potential for Error

Base rates
Primacy effect
Confirmation bias effect
System 1 thinking
Actuarial (statistical) versus clinical prediction
Confabulation
Assumption of dual directional causality
Oversimplification of the data
Misplaced attributions of causality
Bias and self-deception

The first thing to consider is the *base rate* of a condition or behavior, that is, at what rate or how frequently a condition occurs. This is important because when the base rate of a condition is low, the ability to predict or identify the presence of the condition is fraught with difficulty. Let us say, for example, that the base rate of some event, such as Antisocial personality disorder (F60.2), is just over one in 100 (Neumann & Hare, 2008). A central symptom for a person with antisocial personal disorder (ASPD) is disregard for social norms, rules, and obligations (World Health Organization, 1993). Perhaps you work in a sexual offender treatment center and it is your job to interview 100 residents of that center to determine how many of them have ASPD.

This turns out to be an extremely important question, because, for example, many states in the United States have laws that allow the state to keep a sex offender incarcerated even after they have served their sentence for their crime if they are diagnosed with ASPD. Although some studies that have shown that antisocial attitudes are predictive of recidivism in sexual offenders (Hanson & Bussière, 1998), those results are controversial, and the science demonstrating that ASPD is a major contributing factor to sexual offending is lacking (Hatch-Maillette, Scalora, Huss, & Baumgartner, 2001). However, the societal emotion around sexual offenses is such that the science, at least until recently (see the court case, ongoing at the time of this writing, in Minnesota; Serres, 2015), has generally been ignored. So, given this unfortunate circumstance and because of how many state laws are written, your diagnosis of the person may influence whether that person is allowed to return to society or remains incarcerated. It is often difficult for science to gain a toehold when emotions reign. If you are wrong about your diagnosis, it could result in a circumstance in which an individual who should be free may remain incarcerated or a circumstance in which a person who is, in fact, a danger to society may be freed to commit another sexual crime. It is important to note that because the science connecting ASPD and sexual offending is lacking, your failure to diagnose someone as having ASPD is no guarantee that that person will not reoffend, nor is your diagnosis of ASPD a guarantee that they will. Returning to our example of you interviewing 100 residents, if you are prone to thinking that people who do bad things and are at risk to do bad things again should be locked up and the key should be thrown away (not an uncommon perspective in our society), you might well declare all 100 as having ASPD, thereby likely ensuring in some states that all of them will remain incarcerated. If you are more concerned about locking up potentially innocent people, you might be much more conservative in whom you diagnose as having ASPD, which may increase the risk to certain vulnerable people in the society.

For the sake of our example, let us say your job now is to make a prediction about which sex offenders whom you evaluate are likely to reoffend (and, therefore, should remain incarcerated) and which can safely be released. Let us assume for the moment, incorrectly based on the science we have cited but consistent with what many state laws seem to assume (or, at least, lean toward), a perfect correlation between ASPD and future risk of sexual offending, that is, that individuals with ASPD are much more likely to offend again than others without ASPD. On the basis of this set of circumstances, if you state that you believe a sex offender is likely to reoffend or you diagnose that person as having ASPD, you likely are ensuring that that person will remain incarcerated. In our example demonstrating the effects of base rates, it does not matter much whether you predict or merely diagnose. Further, perhaps you are aware of the literature that suggests that the rate of ASPD among sex offenders has been estimated to be in the range of 30% (Borchard, Gnoth, & Schulz, 2003; Motiuk & Porporino, 1992), but you are not aware that the recidivism rate for sexual offenses is likely to be considerably lower than that, as one study found that only 5% (California Department of Corrections and Rehabilitation, 2010) of ASPD and non-ASPD sexual offenders reoffend, and other studies have shown a somewhat higher rate of reoffending, for both ASPD and non-ASPD offenders (cf. Harris & Hanson, 2004). This means that only a minority (even in the Harris & Hanson, 2004, study) of sex offenders will, in fact, reoffend. In reality, because some without ASPD will reoffend, the percentage of ASPD reoffenders may be less than 5%, so the differences in rates may be even more dramatic than initial impressions. So, to continue with the example, you take as your base rate for reoffense 30%, based roughly on the findings by Borchard et al. (2003) and Motiuk and Porporino (1992) and assuming similar to the state laws, that all offenders with ASPD will reoffend, even though the reoffense rate will be even higher, that is, all those with ASPD and some percentage of those without ASPB will reoffend. However, in our example you are being conservative and sticking with the 30%.

All of that leads us to the fundamental question in our hypothesized example: What kinds of prediction accuracies would that lead you to? Let us assume that you are really good at identifying people who are likely to reoffend, regardless of whether their diagnosis is ASPD, so your hit rate (the percentage of those who will reoffend that you identify as reoffenders) with those people is 100% (a very unlikely outcome, by the way, but we are giving you the benefit of the doubt, in this instance). But, being conservative, you have also included some people as reoffenders, who, in reality, will not reoffend, and let us set your hit rate with this category also pretty high, say at 90%.

If the base rate were 30%, your overall accuracy would look as follows. You evaluate 100 sex offenders and you get all of the true positives correct, that is, 30. And because your error rate is pretty low, you correctly identify 29 (rounding up based on the 90% hit rate) of the 30, but of the 70 who will not reoffend, you misidentify seven. So, overall, your accuracy rate is 92%, pretty good (except for the one person you let go who will reoffend and the seven you keep locked up even though they would not reoffend—too bad for them). How would your accuracy compare with someone who randomly assigned people to categories based on statistically probabilities, that is, 30% to the reoffender group and 70% to the nonoffender group, without doing any other screening? Your accuracy is better, but not by as much as one might expect. You accurately classify 92% of the people, and the actuary correctly classifies 84%.

This all assumes, however, an accurate consideration of base rates. What happens if your knowledge of the literature (or your beliefs about sex offenders) leads you to believe that the base rate is 30%, so your classifications remain the same, but the actual base rate is 5%, as in the data from the California Department of Corrections? This is much closer to the case if the actual literature on the correlation between ASPD and risk of sexual offending is followed. In this case, the actuarial classification results in a 90.5% accuracy rate (still not as good as your 92% in the 30% base rate example). However, you still classify 30 of the 100 individuals as high risk. Let us assume you identify all of the bad actors correctly, meaning all five of them. But now you have incorrectly classified 25 people who are not likely to offend as people who should remain incarcerated. That means that your overall accuracy rate has fallen to 75%, well below the result of a random assignment of the actuary, and with pretty dramatic consequences for those 25 people whom you misclassified. (For a discussion of this issue, see Zander, 2005).

To summarize this example, the practical consequence of a lack of consideration of base rates is typically a dramatic overpathologizing of the individual or group under consideration. Table 2.1 (from Greene, 2011, p. 414) provides a guide for the relative accuracy of predictions of a condition (in Greene's table, major depressive disorder) based on the presence of one sign of the condition in the presence of varying levels of base rates. In addition, this discussion assumes the best-case scenario regarding the prediction of any future behavior, about which the empirical data are in fact very discouraging (DeClue, 2013; Yang, Wong, & Coid, 2010).

Another type of base rate should be considered. We have been discussing the base rate of the presence of particular behaviors or characteristics in the population in general and the implications for being able to predict future behaviors accurately if the base rates in the population are low. The other kind of base rate has to do with the degree of variability in behavior within a given individual. Generally, we consider scores or characteristics that are unusual, whether in comparison with other people or for the individual herself/himself, as indicative of a potential problem. However, what if the typical variability in behavior turns out to be quite large, that is, people act in a whole variety of different ways? That would indicate that one cannot simply use the scores (indicating

TABLE 2.1

Effects of Prevalence (Base Rate) on Positive (PPP) and Negative Predictive Power (NPP)

				Prevalence (base rate) = 50%	
Depression Scale 2 (D)	Yes	No	Total	PPP =	350/450 = 77.8%
$T >= 65$	350	100	450	NPP =	400/550 = 72.7%
$T < 65$	150	400	550	Sensitivity =	350/500 = 70.0%
Total	500	500	1000	Specificity =	400/500 = 80.0%
				Prevalence (base rate) = 10%	
Depression Scale 2 (D)	Yes	No	Total	PPP =	70/250 = 28.0%
$T >= 65$	70	180	250	NPP =	720/750 = 96.0%
$T < 65$	30	720	750	Sensitivity =	70/100 = 70.0%
Total	100	900	1000	Specificity =	720/900 = 80.0%
				Prevalence (base rate) = 1%	
Depression Scale 2 (D)	Yes	No	Total	PPP =	7/205 = 3.4%
$T >= 65$	7	198	205	NPP =	792/795 = 99.6%
$T < 65$	3	792	795	Sensitivity =	7/10 = 70.0%
Total	10	990	1000	Specificity =	792/990 = 80.0%

Note. From *The MMPI–2/MMPI–2–RF: An Interpretive Manual* (3rd ed., p. 414), by R. L. Greene, 2011, Boston, MA: Allyn & Bacon. Copyright 2011 by Allyn & Bacon. Reprinted with permission.

variation from some mean) as a basis for concluding that something pathological is going on. It turns out that one study found exactly such variability in test scores within individual test takers (Schretlen, Munro, Anthony, & Pearlson, 2003). One implication that can be drawn from that finding is that conclusions regarding abnormality should not be based on statistical variance by itself but on the degree to which a pattern of results fits recognizable clinical patterns, such as described by ICD–10–CM diagnoses.

Let us take a scenario mentioned briefly above as an example. You are held up at gunpoint in a dark alley. (What possessed you to frequent a dark alley is a whole other issue!) Your response is to behave in a very passive, submissive manner. Although submissive passivity is not a highly unusual behavior in the population as a whole, let us assume that it is for you. Does this statistically unusual behavior therefore constitute a disorder? Given the circumstances, probably not—a message that for psychologists, diagnosis should never occur independent of the context. However, apart from the context, the answer would also be probably not, because passivity is not pathognomonic, that is, by itself reflective of a disorder. Passivity is on a behavioral continuum that may or may not be reflective of a problem. What if your behavior is at the other end of this behavioral continuum, that is, you react with intense aggression in such a way that you do serious bodily damage, and maybe even death, to your assailant? Does that reflect a disorder? In our society, that may be a political question. In a psychological context, it is probably not a disorder if this is the only time in your life you have reacted in that way and you did so only to protect yourself. If, however, it is a behavior that occurs with fairly high statistical frequency for you, it does fit an ICD–10–CM category, such as Antisocial personality disorder (F60.2), or Explosive personality (disorder) coded under Borderline personality disorder (F60.3) or any one of a number of ICD–10–CM diagnoses in Chapter 18, including Hostility (F45.5), Violent behavior (F45.6), State of emotional shock and stress, unspecified (F45.7), or Homicidal ideations (F45.850).

Failing to consider the effects of base rates is not the only error inherent in the process of assessing and diagnosing individuals (for a longer list than we can consider here, see Pope, 2014). The design to organize and understand information is such a powerful motive for humans (Kahneman, 2011; B. Weiner, 1986; see also below) that it leads to number of cognitive errors. One of these errors is the *primacy effect* (Deese & Kaufman, 1957; Murdock, 1962). That is, we as psychologists tend to overvalue the importance of information provided early in the assessment process, to a large degree because we use that information to help us formulate an understanding of the person, which colors our interpretation of data we collect subsequently. That, in turn, leads us to the second of those errors, favoring evidence that supports our thinking and ignoring evidence that conflicts with the conclusions we have already drawn, the *confirmation bias effect* (J. St. B. T. Evans, 1989; Nickerson, 1998). A confirmation bias is the tendency all people have to look for and think about evidence or experiences that confirm their beliefs, because they like being right as opposed to wrong, as opposed to looking for data that contradict their beliefs (Davies, 2003). Why would one want to look for disconfirming data? Because if we do not, we never know when we are wrong. In working with people professionally, that is a big problem. In our experience in dealing with complaints to licensing boards, professionals are more likely to do harm to others because of a lack of consideration of alternative hypotheses than because of evil intent.

Daniel Kahneman (2011), in his wonderful book *Thinking, Fast and Slow*, provides in part a summary of his career-long quest to understand cognitive processes and assumptions. His work, which resulted in a Nobel Prize, suggests that people have two cognitive systems, also constructs. The first is fast *System 1 thinking*, which allows people to react to their environments quickly and efficiently, that is, intuitively. The second system, *System 2 thinking*, involves a deliberate process of considering a variety of data and using analytic abilities to decide what is important and drawing conclusions that are appropriate in any given situation, resulting in the ability to take measured and well-considered suitable action. System 1 develops over time, based on experiences and the connections or associations people make between events that occur together. Thus, it is more a correlational than a causational system, that is, people draw conclusions on the basis of the relationships between events. Its advantage is that it enables people to react quickly and automatically to these events, without the need for expensive (in terms of both time and energy) mental processes or calculations. Sometimes, the speed of responding can be lifesaving. However, System 1 can also lead to errors, because it does not have the ability to evaluate or make judgments about the stimuli to which it reacts. In a psychological assessment situation, System 1 can lead us as psychologists to draw automatic and erroneous conclusions about situations or people we are assessing. One common error is to draw conclusions based on availability to our conscious thinking of events or data, the *availability heuristic* (Kahneman & Tversky, 1972). Thus, for example, because it is easier to think of words that begin with the letter *k* rather than have a *k* as the third letter, people tend to think that more words begin with the letter *k* than have *k* as the third letter, even though it turns out that is not true.

A second common error is what Kahneman and his late collaborator, Amos Tversky, called the *representative heuristic* (Kahneman & Tversky, 1972). Consider the following question from the discussion above: You are doing a psychological assessment on a sex offender. Is that person more likely to have ASPD or not? Most of us psychologists would probably say that the person is more likely to have ASPD than not, because we believe (based on System 1 processes, that is, what we have "picked up" through reading or conversations) that sexual offending is a representative antisocial behavior. The correct answer, however, is no, because we know from the discussion above that the percentage of sex offenders with a diagnosis of ASPD is around 30%, meaning that 70% of sex offenders do not have ASPD. Your System 2 can understand the logic of the argument (we hope), but your System 1 probably concluded ASPD at first, because it relied on quick, automatic conclusions based, in this case, on the representativeness of the data.

Another approach that makes a very similar point is based on Paul Meehl's (1954, 1986) original work on actuarial (statistical) versus clinical prediction (for an excellent review, see Grove, 2005). Meehl essentially showed that using statistical probabilities, one can do a better job of prediction than using clinical information—a sobering thought for all of us psychologists! Meehl's idea, understandably, has been controversial (see Holt, 1958, and Zubin, 1956), given that clinical prediction is the lifeblood of what we as psychologists do, whether in therapy (predicting what will happen in the future based on current circumstances, e.g., a suicide attempt, vs. what will or can happen based on changes that are made in therapy) or in assessment (which often explicitly demands predictions, whether about employability, the effects of disability, the ability to manage one's own affairs, the need for treatment, the likelihood of a convicted felon reoffending, etc.) or even in licensing boards (who is going to be an ethical and competent psychologist) and among faculty/supervisors (what kinds of knowledge and skills are necessary to be an ethical and competent psychologist). However, most subsequent research has provided support for Meehl's original position, whether such research has examined interrater reliability among clinicians, (Goldberg, 1968; P. R. Miller, Dasher, Collins, Griffiths, & Brown, 2001), accuracy in predicting suicidality (G. S. Brown, Jones, Betts, & Wu, 2003), or reviews of the literature on the question of statistical versus clinical prediction itself (Ægisdóttir et al., 2006; Grove, Zald, Lebow, Snitz, & Nelson, 2000).

Research from a very different area of psychology makes a similar point about how people's brains work in two regards. Antonio Damasio (2010), a neurologist who has long grappled with the issues in neuroscience, such as how memories are formed, the role of emotion in decision making, and consciousness, stated that the basic automatic processes (similar to Kahneman's, 2011, System 1) that contribute to people's survival, preexisted their more deliberate side, similar to System 2. The evolutionary progress that enabled people to store images in memory allowed for their more reflective cognitive processes to use those stored images for "effective anticipation of situations, previewing of possible outcomes, navigation of the possible future, and invention of management solutions" (p. 187). This sounds very much like the Kahneman's (2011) System 2 and very much like what a good psychologist should do.

The second contribution from neuroscience proposes that people's brains have a strong need to make sense of experience, to create a coherent whole out of many, sometimes disparate, parts (Damasio, 2010; Frankl, 1963; Proulx & Inzlicht, 2012; Steger, 2012). One of the ways people make sense is to create stories, about themselves and the world in which they live. Stories, which are ubiquitous in various human cultures, create the coherent whole people need. In fact, Damasio (2010) saw the telling of stories as foundational to the core of who people are and how they understand themselves, the subjective sense they have that they are actors in their environment: "Storytelling is something brains do, naturally and implicitly. Implicit storytelling has created our selves, and it should be no surprise that it pervades the entire fabric of human societies and cultures" (p. 311).

However, in telling stories, the details are less important than the whole. As cognitive neuroscientist Michael Gazzaniga (2011) wrote, "Our human brains are driven to infer causality. They are driven to explain events that make sense out of the scattered facts" (p. 77); "facts are great, but not necessary" (p. 88); and "if there is an obvious explanation we accept it. . . . When there is not an obvious explanation, we generate one" (p. 89). What is ultimately important to people is that the stories they tell others and themselves help explain the world they experience and their place in it. Gazzaniga referred to this process as *confabulation*, that is, the concocting of a story that makes sense, even when the facts do not support the story. People are storytellers because making sense out of experiences likely had evolutionary value. Most events do occur for a reason, and understanding that reason helps people cope with those events. So humans' brains are structured in such a way that they look for coherence, even when coherence is not present— or even when the story they tell, the coherence they believe is present, is the wrong story (see also classic experiments by Kelley, 1967; Kleck & Strenta, 1980; and Schachter & Singer, 1962).

An important message for the professional psychologist is that something is fundamental about the ways our brains work that helps us to create a coherent story out of all of the information we gather about the people with whom we work. The good news is that we are able to make sense of the individual events and experiences people tell us about and communicate that sense to others, as well as use that sense to benefit our patients. The bad news is that the stories we create can be dead wrong, although they appear to be logical and realistic (Gottschall, 2012). Coherence is no proof of accuracy. Nor is the amount of information we gather a guarantee of the accuracy of our conclusions, an issue we discuss below. Research has indicated that the more we know about something, the more we can delude ourselves into thinking that what we conclude is accurate (Son & Kornell, 2010). Beware the overly confident psychologist—even psychologists who are also authors sharing their views of how the world is!

Another common error in understanding the causes of events is the *assumption of dual directional causality*. For example, because a person with lung cancer has a very high probability of being a smoker (99%; Dawes, 1988), it is easy and common to assume that smoking is an extremely useful predictor of lung cancer, that is, if a person smokes, she or he is highly likely to get lung cancer. However, actuarial tables indicate that only 10% of smokers get lung cancer. The relevance for this error in psychological diagnoses would be if a particular diagnosis had a high incidence of a particular characteristic—for instance, hallucinations or, perhaps, a high score on the Schizophrenia scale (Scale 8) on the Minnesota Multiphasic Personality Inventory—2 (Butcher, Dahlstrom, Graham, Tellegen, & Kaemmer, 1989)—to believe without additional data that the presence of that characteristic is an indication of the presence of schizophrenia, when, in fact, a person might present with hallucinations or a high Scale 8 score for numerous other reasons. Remember Table 2.1? It depicts a situation in which the presence of one symptom typical of a disorder is used to assume the presence of the disorder in the face of varying base rates.

Another error we believe is important to mention is *oversimplification of data*. We started this discussion with the description of the massive amount of data of varying sorts that a clinician gathers during an assessment process. Even if we, as psychologists, are aware of the dangers of relying too strongly on Kahneman's (2011) System 1 in our deliberations, it is still the case that the data we gather are so voluminous that we have to choose. We have to identify what we think are the most important facts or factors. We have to categorize so that we can keep track of and make sense of the disparate bits of information we receive. We have to draw connections between variables whenever possible to draw necessary conclusions and to make sense out of separate bits of information. In the process of engaging in those rather complex cognitive processes, we also run the risk of leaving out important data, especially data that do not fit our developing theories or conceptualizations of the person (recall the primacy and confirmation bias effects). We see what we expect to see and do not see what we do not expect to see. That leads us to not follow up on threads that might be important. However, we are often not even aware of our error. So, we package the information in ways that make it manageable and intelligible but thereby miss important keys or factors and overvalue other factors that we think explain what they might not explain. We need to continuously guard against becoming overconfident with the data we possess and the conclusions we draw.

Because of our need to understand and categorize, we have a tendency to try to attribute causality to events without clear causality, referred to as *misplaced attributions of causality*. If we try to make sense out of complex situations, to provide order where little order exists, by making predictions about how things are likely to go in the future, we run the risk of trying to fit random data (noise) into our conceptualizations, which may result in garbage in, garbage out (Silver, 2012), leading to unsupported conclusions and predictions. Psychologists are often asked to provide a glimpse into the future—what treatment will work with this person, is that person likely to continue to act abnormally, is this person likely to be a danger to self or others? Our predictions can even be erroneous when they are based on common clinical lore: The best predictor of future behavior is past behavior. Although that is very often true, such predictions assume that circumstances in the future will be the same as they were in the past, when in fact things sometimes change.

The fundamental argument we are making here is that it is crucial for psychologists to be intentional, deliberate, and thoughtful in what we do. Human brains are structured in such a way that unconscious, automatic processes will take over whatever tasks they can, to allow our conscious minds to focus on more salient or more challenging aspects of our environments. Allowing our unconscious sway over psychological decision making, however, comes with a risk that we will fall into the variety of cognitive errors we have discussed above. To quote Damasio (2010) again, "We cannot run our kind of life, in the physical and social environments that have become the human habitat, without reflective, conscious deliberation" (p. 288). Further, to paraphrase a favored saying of a high-school teacher friend of one of us, "The person who fails to read directions gives up the advantage she or he has over the illiterate." We would say, the psychologist who fails to use a deliberate, intentional, scientific approach to data gives up the advantage she or he has over the other creatures in the animal kingdom. As Damasio (2010) stated, "Taking the time to analyze facts, to evaluate the outcome of decisions, and to ponder the emotional results of those decisions is the path to building a practical guide otherwise known as wisdom" (p. 297).

Perhaps the most serious error to which humans are prone is the ease with which we can deceive not only others but also ourselves. We are good at *self-deception*. Kahneman (2011) stated it this way: We have an "almost unlimited ability to ignore our ignorance" (p. 201). Carol Tavris and Elliot Aronson (2007), in their very readable and insightful book *Mistakes Were*

Made (But Not by Me), discussed our seemingly never-ending abilities to convince ourselves that our errors are not errors at all, but justified and based correctly on the information available.[1] Michael Gazzaniga (2011), from a neuropsychological perspective, made the further point that all of our conscious conclusions are merely post hoc explanations or rationalizations for what our brains have already decided at a subconscious level. One form of such an error is the assumption that as professionals, we are objective and without bias. The reality is that we all have biases involving preconceptions. To ignore our biases or to pretend that they do not exist is to open ourselves to the very biases we pretend not to have by viewing the hypotheses we develop—and should develop—as fact, rather than as hypotheses that need to be tested by comparisons with collected data. This potential for bias, particularly in a context in which a clinician has to make decisions about which data to discard and which to privilege and pursue, is a major reason that a diagnostic system like the ICD–10–CM is so helpful. Knowing how symptoms group together in diagnostic categories enables psychologists to focus our attention on elements of the person's history and present functioning that have the highest probability of providing useful information to answer the referral questions. We now turn to that process of collecting and considering data to answer specific questions.

---

[1]*Mistakes Were Made (But Not by Me)* is largely a modern application of cognitive consistency theories (see Abelson et al., 1968) generally and cognitive dissonance theory (Festinger, 1957) more specifically.

Conducting an Assessment and Making a Diagnosis

3

n this chapter, we describe the challenges involved in the process of deciding on a diagnosis for the specific individuals with whom we work. In Chapter 2, we described the complexities and pitfalls of diagnosis and the necessity of providing diagnoses, but we did not explore how a psychologist goes about the process of deciding on a diagnosis. How does a psychologist ensure, as best as he or she can, that the process that leads to a diagnosis, using the Clinical Modification of the *International Statistical Classification of Diseases and Related Health Problems* (ICD–10–CM; National Center for Health Statistics, 2015), is thorough, objective, and accurate?

Theodore Millon (1969) suggested that clinical analysis involves four steps:

(a) a survey of the patient's current clinical picture, (b) tracing the developmental influences which shaped the problem, (c) constructing a model or syndrome representing the central features of the patient's pathology, and (d) formulating a remedial plan for management and therapy. (p. 110)

http://dx.doi.org/10.1037/14778-004
A Student's Guide to Assessment and Diagnosis Using the ICD–10–CM: Psychological and Behavioral Conditions, by J. Schaffer and E. Rodolfa

More recently, Bram and Peebles (2014) described variations on this process in their discussion of psychological testing, but across the years and regardless of the goals, the steps remain basically the same: (a) collect data, including information about developmental influences; (b) make sense of the data; and (c) develop an intervention or disposition plan.

Collecting Data

The first phase involves collecting the data necessary for the purposes of the psychological service being provided. As we discuss more fully later, the ICD–10–CM can be of assistance in the data collection process to help psychologists focus on the relevant symptoms and signs for each disorder.

The data collection process begins with a plan to gather information, both the signs (objective data) observed during the interview and the symptoms (subjective experiences) described by the patient. As the psychologist interacts with the patient, a plan is refined, focusing on the additional data needed and the means by which those data will be collected. The psychologist has five major methods to acquire psychological data, which we summarize in Exhibit 3.1: (a) clinical interview, (b) record review, (c) behavioral observations, (d) psychological testing, and (e) collateral interviews.

CLINICAL INTERVIEW

A clinical interview provides both current and historical information. See Exhibit 3.2 for the areas it would be helpful to cover during an inter-

---

EXHIBIT 3.1

Major Sources of Psychological Data

Clinical interview: Extensive interview of the current functioning and history of the evaluee, covering some or all of the topics below

Record review: Reviewing and evaluating records from other mental health and health professionals, schools, employers, legal records, and other relevant professional records

Behavioral observations: All observations of the evaluee's behavior during the interview and testing, including a formal mental status examination, if appropriate

Psychological testing: Use of standardized psychological tests that are valid for the purpose being used

Collateral interviews: When appropriate, interviews with others who may know the evaluee well (including other professionals, friends, parents, teachers, employers)

EXHIBIT 3.2

Outline of Interview Protocol

1. Reason for referral
2. Family-of-origin background
3. Interpersonal relationships
4. Educational background
5. Vocational history
6. Interests/hobbies
7. Subjective strengths/weaknesses
8. Other important life events/traumatic experiences
9. Current psychological state
10. Legal history
11. Medical history
12. Chemical use
13. Daily activities
14. Current functioning
15. Personal goals

view. In addition to having such an outline as a template, the interplay between data gathering, diagnostic impression, and diagnostic hypothesis from the ICD–10–CM, informed by a text like the *Blue Book* (World Health Organization, 1993) or a text such as those suggested in Chapter 10 (this volume), also helps you to focus your interview questions. In other words, our perspective is that an interview will not and should not simply follow in rote fashion an outline such as found in Exhibit 3.2 but should be informed by the specific questions whose answers you are seeking. Relying on the ICD–10–CM helps you to formulate those specific questions. The interplay between the data gathered and the diagnostic possibilities should be ongoing, with the data informing the differential diagnoses and the diagnoses informing the additional data that need to be gathered. A structured interview such as the Structured Clinical Interview for *DSM–5* (First, Williams, Karg, & Spitzer, 2015) can also be helpful in focusing interview questions on specific diagnostic categories. The ICD–10–CM provides a basis for knowing better what type of data is important to gather not just during the interview but also in the other methods of data collection discussed below.

How extensive the interview needs to be will depend on the purposes of the assessment and the rights to privacy. The more impact the assessment is likely to have on a person's life, the more extensive the interview should generally be and the more likely one will need to gather most or all of the information listed by Exhibit 3.2. Unless the questions are asked, a psychologist cannot know for certain what information should be gathered and how it might be relevant to the assessment. Covering in some detail the topics contained in Exhibit 3.2, plus those questions specific to the ICD–10–CM diagnostic possibilities, an interview normally will take from 3 to 7 hours, depending very much on the complexity of the clinical situation and the talkativeness of the evaluee. With the extensive gathering of personal information, consideration for inclusion in the record must be balanced, however, with the evaluee's right to privacy. The ethics codes of both the American Psychological Association (APA, 2010; 4.04a) and the Canadian Psychological Association (2000; I, 37) state that only that information "germane to the purpose" of the assessment should be collected. The evaluee may have some event or behavior in the past that has nothing to do with the reasons for the assessment but that may compromise her or his well-being or cause embarrassment. The psychologist should be sensitive to such concerns and work to maintain a balance between respecting the individual's right to privacy, on the one hand, and gathering all of the information necessary for a valid assessment, on the other. This is an area in which supervision or consultation is especially warranted and helpful. The specific question is, can the referral questions be answered fully without providing this piece of information?

RECORDS

Psychological, medical, school, work, and/or legal records can provide useful information. Records may be available at the first interview, either supplied by the referral source or previous records in a clinic, if the patient has received prior health services. Sometimes, helpful records will need to be requested from relevant providers. If such records are needed, it will be necessary to secure a release of information to request the records (see further discussion in Chapter 8, this volume).

BEHAVIORAL OBSERVATION

Behavioral observation includes all observations of the behaviors and style of the interviewee, during the interview and in other contexts, such as interacting with the psychologist's office staff, which can provide very useful insights. Behavioral observations include how a person comports himself or herself, facial expressions, and how information is conveyed (i.e., tone of voice, emphasis, and apparent emotional reactions). Such observations are often referred to as the *mental status examination*, which includes observations of the person's behavior and an estimate of level of cognitive functioning, that is, a rough estimate of the integrity of the individual's brain. Exhibit 3.3 provides an overview of the components of a mental status examination.

Because such external observations include conclusions about what is happening internally with a person, both emotionally and cognitively, on the basis of external behaviors, one should be very cautious about using them to draw conclusions, as opposed to simply reporting the observa-

> ### EXHIBIT 3.3
>
> **Mental Status Examination Overview**
>
> - Basic grooming and hygiene
> - Gait and motor coordination
> - Interview behavior and manner
> - Interpersonal characteristics and approach to assessment
> - Behavioral interactions
> - Speech
> - Expressive language
> - Mood and affect
> - General feelings most days
> - Feelings expressed during the interview
> - Establishing rapport
> - Behavioral expression of emotions
> - Thought processes and content/orientation
> - Orientation
> - Alertness
> - Coherence
> - Concentration and attention
> - Hallucinations and delusions
> - Judgment and insight

tions. For example, one could describe the person as talking with a loud voice, using dramatic words (e.g., expletives), and frowning, or as having difficulty remembering information or tracking the questions posed. However, one could not necessarily conclude that the person is angry, or even more so, that the person has a propensity toward violence or that the person is brain damaged. Behavioral observations can also be considered to include the clinician's own reaction to the evaluee. Given the biases that can be part of our responses to a variety of stimuli, the problems inherent in our emotional reactions to those we work with professionally is apparent. However, those reactions can also provide useful clinical information (see Colli, Tanzilli, Dimaggio, & Lingiardi, 2014). Damasio (1994, 2000) has long argued that emotions are an important part of decision making. In this context, your emotional reactions to people with whom you work professionally is one important source of information and is to be compared with the other sources of information discussed here. The role of such reactions should be a part of the supervision every reader of this book has had or will have.

PSYCHOLOGICAL TESTING

Psychological testing is an area that historically has been unique to psychologists. In the earlier days of clinical psychology, psychological testing was the primary activity of professional psychologists, and it continues to be the second most common professional service offered by psychologists, next to psychotherapy (Weiner, 2013). The use of psychological tests requires a number of considerations: errors, objectivity, validity, bias, fit, added value, and accuracy. The following discussion examines each of these issues in turn.

One primary reason we as psychologists use tests is because we are concerned about the errors inherent in other kinds of data we collect, which are in part dependent on the perspectives and approaches of the psychologist, or of others, in the cases of records and collateral interviews. Psychological test data, on the other hand, are independent of us and so can be used as a more objective measure of the accuracy of our developing theories of the person we are evaluating. Ample studies demonstrate the reliability and validity of psychological tests (see Meyer et al., 2001). That gives psychological testing a unique role in our gathering of relevant information. Psychologists use literally hundreds of tests. Professional neuropsychologists, who use tests as a primary assessment tool, were surveyed a few years ago to determine which tests are used most often. The Wechsler tests (Wechsler, 2008, 2014), among cognitive measures, and the Minnesota Multiphasic Personality Inventory—2 (MMPI-2; Butcher, Dahlstrom, Graham, Tellegen, & Kaemmer, 1989), among personality measures, were found to be the most frequently used (Rabin, Barr, & Burton, 2005). A recent survey of faculty who teach assessment techniques found training occurred most frequently with these same tests (Ready & Veague, 2014).

Two important criteria guide psychologists in choosing specific tests for use in an assessment, regardless of whether the evaluation process is formal (e.g., in response to a referral from another professional or a court and involving the writing of a formal report) or informal (e.g., a first step in providing psychotherapy, involving collecting only as much data as reasonable or necessary and, usually, without a written report). The first criterion is whether a test being used has been shown empirically to be valid and reliable for the purposes and with the population for which it is to be used. In other words, for the person you are assessing, does the test actually measure what it is you want it to measure? The answer to that question depends on the standardization data. When the test was developed for use with a certain group of people, the test is given to a representative sample from that group and data collected about how they perform. Those data then serve as the norms, the criteria against which the person you are testing is compared. If the person you are assessing does not bear substantial resemblance to the normative sample[1] (the definition of what substantial resemblance requires is not

---

[1]There is no definitive definition of what *substantial resemblance* requires—another instance in which psychology is also an art based on clinical judgment, as well as a science based on empirical data.

definitive—another instance in which psychology is also an art based on clinical judgment, as well as a science based on empirical data), then you will have no idea how your evaluee should perform on the test and no way of interpreting the results of the test. For example, the Wechsler Adult Intelligence Scale—IV (WAIS–IV; Wechsler, 2008) has been well validated as a measure of intelligence with English-speaking people, but it is not a good choice for someone who does not speak English or does not speak English fluently. Without further empirical data, researchers would have no idea how a person who does not speak English fluently should do on the WAIS–IV, even though it is a well-validated test. So, although researchers know what an IQ of 100 means in the normative sample, they have no idea what it means with a group different from the normative sample. Further, the WAIS–IV is not intended as a measure of personality, although Wechsler tests were once used in that way (Rapaport, Gill, & Schafer, 1974). Thus, a test should be used only for the specific purpose for which it was designed. A more realistic example these days is, perhaps, the use of the MMPI–2 for questions of employment. That is, should the MMPI–2 be used as a screening test to determine whether a person will be a good employee? Certainly, the MMPI (Hathaway & McKinley, 1942) and, subsequently, the MMPI–2, were not developed with employment considerations in mind. They were developed as a means of determining who was experiencing a major psychological dysfunction and who is likely to need hospitalization. However, thousands of studies have been done on the MMPI and the MMPI–2, and studies have been done that standardize the use of the MMPI–2 in specific employment contexts (e.g., police officers; Butcher, Ones & Cullen, 2006; Detrick, Chibnall, & Rosso, 2001; Sellbom, Fischler, & Ben-Porath, 2007). As a test user who has been trained in the MMPI–2, you should also know the literature well enough to determine whether norms for this test, or any test, have been developed for the person you are asked to assess, or if you are asked to assess someone different from people you have previously assessed, you should search the empirical literature to see what studies have been done (see additional discussion of this general issue in Chapter 7, this volume).

Another issue to consider in using psychological tests is assessor error. We made the statement above that psychological test data are unique and valuable because they provide information that is independent of us as the examiner. A more accurate statement would be that they are independent of us—except when they're not! In cases of assessor bias[2] in the use of tests, as well as in the interpretation of observed behaviors (Hoyt & Kerns, 1999; Miller, Rufino, Boccaccini, Jackson,

---

[2]*Assessor bias* is the lack of objectivity in the mental health professional that occurs during the process of collecting and evaluating assessment data.

& Murrie, 2011). A primary risk to consider is the use of nonstandard means of administration and test scoring. Such errors are particularly likely in the Wechsler tests (Kaufman & Lichtenberger, 2006) but are also possible with straightforward self-report tests, such as the MMPI–2 if nonstandard administrations are used (Butcher, Graham, & Ben-Porath, 1995). An additional problem is that assessor error is typically not reported in testing manuals (McDermott, Watkins, & Rhoad, 2014). The possibility of such errors should emphasize the importance of standard use of tests and of some humility in our use of any kind of data.

The second criterion, related to the first, is that the tests used constitute a "battery" rather than a "pile" of tests (T. Boll, personal communication, October 15, 1976). That is, tests should be chosen for a specific purpose, to measure a specific type of characteristic or ability, and multiple tests should be chosen to complement each other, that is, to provide different types of information or to provide some degree of corroboration for other tests and other sources of information, all of which are intended to fit the purposes of the assessment. Thus, a test should be used only if it will provide needed or helpful information. In other words, the exact questions meant to be answered by the assessment in general, and the testing specifically, should be determined ahead of time and a decision made about the kinds of tests that together will provide reliable and valid answers to those questions. Obviously, this means that you have to have a clear idea of what the referral question is—sometimes a much more difficult task than is initially obvious. Not infrequently, the psychologist may have to engage in a training process with referral sources, helping them to ask the right kinds of questions, with the understanding that they are much more likely to get their questions answered in a helpful and accurate way if the psychologist knows what the questions are. The alternative to a battery, the pile of tests, constitutes using a variety of tests because the clinician is acquainted with them and knows what they mean, but in a specific clinical context has no particular thought about why one test rather than another. A pile of tests will produce a pile of data, the meaning of which is likely to be difficult or impossible to determine.

We believe that psychological testing should be used in formal assessments when possible (i.e., whenever a test is reliable and valid for the purposes of the assessment and resources allow), because of the uniqueness the data testing provides, that is, the data from testing are like no other data psychologists obtain in that they are less dependent on the subjectivity of the observer. The other reason is that many psychological tests included what are called *embedded measures of dissimulation*, that is, measures of whether the test taker is approaching the test in an open and honest manner, or conversely, whether he or she is exaggerating or underreporting problems, or perhaps, some combination of those two (depending on the nature and social acceptability of the problems). All people, including psychologists, are notoriously ineffective in judging people's honesty by observation alone (Hurd & Noller, 1988). So, the embedded measures are some of the only objective ways we psychologists have of determining whether the assessment overall of the individual is likely to be accurate and valid, based on the person's approach to the assessment process.

Many in the field do not agree that testing should typically be used, however (see, e.g., Jackson et al., 2011; Walfish, Vance, & Fabricatore, 2007). Psychological tests are less frequently used as part of a treatment planning process during psychotherapy, both because insurance companies are less inclined to reimburse for testing in therapy and because the focus of therapy should primarily be on the needs and goals of the patient, rather than the needs of the psychologist to gather complete information. Nevertheless, when psychologists use psychological tests as part of the provision of psychotherapy, tests can provide helpful information because they sample a different type of behavior than that observed in an intake interview and ongoing data gathering in therapy. One primary question in a therapy context is whether a sufficient amount of additional useful information is likely to be obtained through the use of tests to justify the additional expense in both time and money. We do want to emphasize that a process of assessment, whether including the use of tests or not, is an essential component of all psychotherapy. One cannot help another person deal with problems without an understanding of the problems and of the person who exhibits those problems. John Hunsley (2007) makes this point in arguing convincingly that skill in assessment is essential to being able to engage in evidence-based practice.

COLLATERAL INTERVIEWS

Collateral interviews are conducted with persons other than the individual being evaluated who might be able to provide additional information from a different perspective (e.g., family members, teachers, employers, friends). Collateral interviews are common in some forensic assessment contexts and less common as part of a treatment planning procedure for psychotherapy, except interviewing family members when the patient is a minor.

An important consideration in doing collateral interviews is privacy. In most states, the communications between a psychologist and a client are confidential and cannot be passed on to others. By its nature, doing a collateral interview means breaking confidentiality by letting the collateral interviewee know that the evaluee is being assessed. Most often, the privacy considerations override the value of the additional information in a psychotherapy context, although collateral interviews could proceed with the consent of the person (see Chapter 8, this volume, for a more complete discussion of informed consent). In a forensic context, someone's freedom or employment or monetary compensation or some other fairly significant outcome may provide a strong enough basis for gathering the information that the patient or evaluee (or, sometimes, a court) will decide that privacy is not a prohibitive factor. For further consideration of some of the ethical issues involved in conducting an assessment, see Chapter 7, this volume; APA (2010); and Sattler and Schaffer (2014).

As discussed above, the precise procedures used to gather data will depend on the purposes and the context of the assessment. It is important to use procedures and sources of data that are adequate to the conclusions provided (see APA, 2010, Section 9.01). To quote from APA's (2013) *Specialty Guidelines for Forensic Psychology*:

> Forensic practitioners ordinarily avoid relying solely on one source of data, and corroborate important data whenever feasible. . . . When relying upon data that have not been corroborated, forensic practitioners seek to make known . . . any associated strengths and limitations, and the reasons for relying upon the data. (p. 15)

These guidelines are useful for forensic psychologists as well as all psychologists who provide nonforensic psychological testing.

You might ask yourself two additional questions as you think about what kinds of data are necessary for your assessment and how you should go about collecting those data: What are the consequences to the evaluee of your being wrong in your assessment of him or her (either by misidentifying the problems present or by either over- or understating the problems), and what implications does that have for how comprehensive and varied your data should be? Remember that during your experiential training, you will have supervisors who will assist you with these complex questions.

In sum, the psychologist gathers information that is appropriate to the purpose and goals of the assessment. She or he is also clear and transparent about procedures, purposes, and sources of data, and discusses the limitations of the sources of data and procedures used in the assessment process.

Making Sense of the Data

Once we have significant amounts of data, we return to our starting point, namely, how to make sense out of all of that information. We must sort through all of the bits of data we have to draw appropriate conclusions and make helpful recommendations without leaving out important information or being biased in the data we emphasize. A number of guidelines can help us psychologists accomplish that goal.

It is important that no information is ignored. In fact, information that seems not to fit may be especially useful, and it requires careful consideration. With respect to all data obtained, the clinician should ask, Could this be important? Does this information provides insight into the evaluee's experience and the ICD–10–CM diagnostic possibilities? Is there something about this information that can shape or reshape the hypotheses and conclusions I have? And, beyond that, should the information be included in a report or is it unimportant enough, or private enough, to be excluded? Not all information can or should be included or the outcome (whether a written or verbal report) would be so voluminous as to be unusable.

Two significant strategies can help a psychologist make decisions about the inclusion or exclusion of data. First, it is important not to draw conclusions or formulate perspectives too early in the process, which is nearly guaranteed to eliminate viable alternatives that might be helpful—and accurate. One good strategy is to wait to draw conclusions until the end of the process, having pulled together and reviewed all of the data relevant enough to be included in the report, enabling you to consider carefully all of the information you have.

Second, an essential aspect of the process of conducting a psychological assessment is to look for disconfirming evidence. That is, as one begins to draw tentative conclusions and form an overall conceptualization of what the important factors are in the assessment of a particular person, one should very intentionally and actively look for data, from all sources of collected information, that may provide alternative perspectives. With regard to a particular formulation, ask yourself whether any information disagrees with that formulation or provides an alternative viewpoint. Competence in engaging in psychological assessment requires that one be thorough and brutally honest in seeking disconfirming evidence.

When one finds disconfirming information, which is virtually always present in any assessment, what does one do with it? Here, rules are hard to come by because the answer to the question will always depend on the nature of the information available. And, this is where experience with dealing with complex data is particularly helpful. A first answer is to seek consultation or supervision for help. In the final analysis, the formulations and conclusions one draws and the degree of confidence one can place in those formulations and conclusions will depend upon how much the various sources of data agree, that is, where the data converge. If multiple sources of data all point in the same direction and very little information suggests an alternative conceptualization, one can present conclusions with a fair degree of confidence in their accuracy. When there is disagreement in the information gathered, one option is to attempt to gather additional information to resolve the discrepancies, but if one has all the data possible or reasonably available, one goes with the conclusions that seem to agree most with the preponderance of the data and acknowledge that one's confidence in those conclusions is lower. One should state the level of confidence openly and clearly in the report.

Last, no assessment and no assessment procedure or technique, whether test or interview or records from others, will be perfectly reliable and valid. With a test, the evaluee of a given assessment and the population on which the test was standardized will never exactly correspond. With an interview, a variety of factors can influence how much the individual reveals about herself or himself, including variability from day to day in mood or outlook, the nature of the professional relationship, and the evaluee's understanding or interpretation of the questions posed. In addition, every psychologist, regardless of how expert or how experienced, has limits to his or her ability to understand in a comprehensive manner the experiences and viewpoints being shared by the patient. With records or other information from others about the evaluee, the other person's own biases and perspective may color interpretations and conclusions. Thus, one should approach all data with due skepticism and remember that the process of drawing conclusions about a person involves comparing and contrasting all of the information collected.

To summarize, the process a psychologist follows when conducting a psychological assessment is based on the scientific methodology of hypothesis generation and hypothesis testing. This methodology starts at the very beginning of the assessment process. When one receives a referral, it is desirable to obtain a certain amount of patient information, along with the specific questions that the referral source would like answered. From the initial request for an assessment, the psychologist begins to formulate some hypotheses about what is occurring and the sources of information that might provide insight. At this point in the process, those hypotheses are a very long way away from conclusions. Rather, they are pathways to guiding the process of collecting specific information.

Developing an Intervention or Disposition Plan

Once the available, relevant information is gathered, one consciously and intentionally uses the scientific methodology a second time, to form coherent explanatory conceptualizations about the person and develop appropriate conclusions. To accomplish this, one begins by formulating hypotheses about possible alternatives. This is another point at which reliance on the ICD–10–CM can be especially helpful. Which diagnostic possibilities have you considered, and how do those diagnoses help you think about what possible alternative explanations help tell a story that is not only coherent but also fits the data? We consider in much more detail in the next chapter how to think about diagnostic possibilities and implications. The next step is to review all of the data that have been collected to assess the support or lack of support for each hypothesis. This process can lead to additional questions that might be pursued by seeking more records, conducting more interviews, or administering more psychological tests, depending on the goals of the assessment. Once all of the necessary and reasonably available data has been collected, one weighs and considers the data and draws conclusions with the appropriate level of confidence. That weighing of the data involves looking for convergence within the data, that is, consistent support from the data for previously developed hypotheses, and comparing the developing conclusions with those hypotheses, from the various sources of data and from the objective diagnostic categories of the ICD–10–CM, to ensure that you have adequately considered the data from sufficient vantage points to know that your conclusions are not only unbiased but also thorough.

This process of evaluating data and reaching conclusions can be both simplified and complicated if the person you are assessing has had previous contact with a mental health professional and comes to you with an ICD–10–CM diagnosis. The process is simplified in that the potential range of diagnostic and assessment options may be narrowed. The previous diagnosis provides you with information regarding what the other mental health professional saw as important and noteworthy. That type of communication from one professional to another is a major reason for diagnosis. The data communicated to you by the diagnosis should be considered carefully. However, it can also be complicated by the increased chance of bias, in this case by narrowing the range of options too much by looking only at those factors emphasized by the other professional. Every psychologist has the ethical and fiduciary duty to consider carefully all of the data available and to make an independent judgment of what data are important, how they fit together, and to which conclusions they lead. Again, using the ICD–10–CM as an objective backdrop assists us in navigating that process. That is, by comparing the information you have with the ICD–10–CM diagnoses and thinking through carefully what the diagnosis means, you can guard against cherry-picking only those data that support your hypotheses.

It is helpful in this process to remember the importance of base rates and to question, once again, the value and accuracy of your data in drawing conclusions in answer to the referral questions for the particular individual. The following three steps can help you decide on the conclusions you draw:

1. "Anchor your judgment of the probability of an outcome on a plausible base rate" (Kahneman, 2011, p. 154).
2. "Question the diagnosticity of your evidence" (Kahneman, 2011, p. 154).
3. In the absence of strong and consistent evidence of your initial prediction, regress your predictions toward the mean (for an excellent and accessible video on regression to the mean, see Schneider, 2013).

This last point means that if you are about to draw a conclusion that is somewhat unusual, (i.e., out of the typical range of behaviors for most human beings), with some degree of disconfirming evidence, consider a conclusion that is less extreme, such as a less severe form of a disorder or, even, a characteristic that is unusual but not pathological.[3] In ICD–10–CM terms, consider instead of an F code (Chapter 5), an R code (signs and symptoms in Chapter 18) or Z code (factors influencing health status in Chapter 21).

This may or may not be the end of your task. If you have been asked to do an assessment only (see the cases in Chapters 4 and 5), then once you have satisfied yourself by carefully considering the data and taken into account the errors you can make in drawing conclusions, your only remaining task is writing a report to share your thinking and conclusions with the referral source. The issues involved in writing a report are beyond the scope of this book, but multiple resources are available for you (see those listed in Chapter 10 for a beginning). If the assessment you have conducted is for the purposes of providing some type of intervention (usually, but not always psychotherapy—it could also be primarily educational or consultation with some other entity), then an additional methodology should be considered in getting from your data and conclusions to the specific interventions that are appropriate. It is that process that provides our focus in Chapter 9.

---

[3]For purposes of this discussion, we define *out of the typical range* as at least one standard deviation away from the mean, which by definition would include all mental health diagnostic categories.

Using the ICD–10–CM

Case 1—Lynn

4

I n the next three chapters, we discuss three examples of assessing and diagnosing using the Clinical Modification of the *International Statistical Classification of Diseases and Related Health Problems* (ICD–10–CM; National Center for Health Statistics, 2015). We have created cases to reflect the referrals psychologists receive, the variety of clinical content, and the range of professional issues psychologists confront. We hope that focusing on these cases helps us and you, the reader, be on the same page, so to speak, in considering clinical, ethical, and risk management issues. The cases are either completely invented, based on our experiences, or are based on one or more real cases but with enough information changed or invented that there is no possibility of identifying one of the patients as a real person (see the American Psychological Association, 2010, *Ethical Principles of Psychologists and Code of Conduct*, Ethical Standard 4.07). The cases are used, further, as the basis for exploring ethical issues raised in clinical practice in Chapter 7, the ways of minimizing risks in practice in Chapter 8, and taking steps toward disposition in Chapter 9.

http://dx.doi.org/10.1037/14778-005
A Student's Guide to Assessment and Diagnosis Using the ICD–10–CM: Psychological and Behavioral Conditions, by J. Schaffer and E. Rodolfa

These cases were developed to provide you a common set of circumstances to explore diagnostic, ethical, risk management, and dispositional considerations. They are meant to be illustrative rather than definitive. That is, they are not intended to cover all or any specific portion of the crucial issues involved in assessment. Rather, we use them to provide some common ground for you to consider some of the issues we believe are important in the process of psychological assessment.

In Chapters 2 and 3, we discussed, in some detail, issues related to the process of engaging in a psychological assessment, and we presented in broad terms the types of data and thinking involved in assessment. In Chapters 4, 5, and 6, in the context of the three cases, we consider in more detail the thinking process a psychologist uses in understanding the needs and perspectives of a patient, what data are needed and why, how to develop appropriate diagnostic hypotheses using the ICD–10–CM, and generally, how to competently conduct an objective assessment of your patient.

Another note on our methodology here: We used the *Blue Book* (World Health Organization [WHO], 1993), a companion volume to the ICD–10–CM, which is a classification system rather than a diagnostic manual. We decided to use the *Blue Book* not because it is the best or most recent diagnostic manual available but because it is readily available online for the reader and provides us with a common text to refer to, in addition to its specificity to the ICD–10–CM. The actual diagnostic manual you decide to use with your own cases may well depend on the texts your professor has assigned for use in your coursework in psychopathology. We also provide some suggested psychopathology texts in Chapter 10.

The Case: Lynn

The following assessment was conducted by you, a doctoral student. You are currently enrolled in your second assessment course and as a course requirement need to complete a recently assigned battery of tests, including the Minnesota Multiphasic Personality Inventory—2 (Butcher, Dahlstrom, Graham, Tellegen, & Kaemmer, 1989), the Millon Clinical Multiaxial Inventory—III (Millon, 2006) and the Stanford–Binet Intelligence Scale (fifth ed.; Roid, 2003), three very commonly used tests of psychological and intellectual functioning. With this assignment in mind, you interviewed and tested the following individual and wrote a report.

PRESENTING CONCERN

At the time of the interview, Lynn was a 25-year-old, single, European American woman. She was living alone and had a good job working as a loan officer at a local bank.

She was referred to the community service agency by her sister, with encouragement from the president of the bank. Lynn reported that her sister has been concerned that Lynn had not been herself for the past few weeks and that her boss was concerned that her work productivity had decreased. Lynn described a growing sense of dread that began soon after her mother died of natural causes about two months ago. She hoped that therapy might be useful to help her understand and change her behavior. You received a written request from the bank president for updates on Lynn's condition and progress, with a focus on whether her job performance was likely to improve in the near future.

RELEVANT HISTORY

Lynn reported a desire to stay at home but said, "I drag myself out of the house to work every day." She found herself worried about going out of her home and did not believe that she was able to concentrate and focus on her work very effectively. She had found herself behind in writing reports at work, and her clients were beginning to complain to her manager. She believed that she was building a good career, was financially stable, and she was proud of her accomplishments but had become worried that she might lose her job.

After their father was killed in a head-on automobile accident with a drunk driver when Lynn was 6 years old, she and her sister were raised by their mother. As a result of the accident, the family received a significant amount of money from life insurance that helped support them. Her mother worked as a real estate agent, which provided the primary financial support for the family. Lynn reported that she was very close to her mother and relied on her for support and advice. She also described a positive supportive relationship with her sister, who lived approximately 900 miles away with her husband and two children, ages 2 and 4.

Lynn was in a 2-year relationship that ended approximately five months ago. She stated that she and her former partner had discussed marriage but that he met someone when he was out with "the boys" and had an affair. He ended the relationship, and then she found out about the affair from a friend of her former boyfriend. Lynn felt betrayed and reported feeling very cautious about meeting men. She had not dated since her relationship ended.

Lynn had a few close friends who lived fairly close to her. She reported that all had "checked in" with her because they had noticed the changes in her behavior and feelings over the past month, but sometimes she thought they were pushing too hard for her to seek help. She did appreciate their concern but felt their focus on her welfare was excessive and hoped they would stop pushing her. But she was unable to tell them to reduce their encouragement because she did not want to offend them.

She used to exercise regularly and felt that she was in good shape. But during the past few weeks, rather than exercising daily as was her past practice, Lynn had been exercising considerably less frequently. On some occasions she had difficulty catching her breath, even when she had not been working out for a long time. She indicated that she usually has a physical exam once a year and that her last one, about 11 months ago, found her to be in good health.

After her mother's death, Lynn began drinking at least one glass of wine a night and on some nights, two or three glasses "to take the edge off." Up until then, her use of alcohol had been limited. She reported that she did not use street drugs and was not taking any medications.

Lynn reported that her mother took her to therapy immediately after her father died. She attended only a few sessions and did not believe it was helpful, although she could not remember much about the experience. As a result, as Lynn began the interview, she expressed concern that therapy might not help her at this point.

CURRENT FUNCTIONING/MENTAL STATUS

Presentation

Lynn was of average height and weight. She appeared healthy, except for a bandage on her right hand, which she described as an accidental cut on her palm while cooking recently. She was dressed in a gray and black suit, as she reported coming to the session immediately from work. She indicated that she usually dresses casually in jeans and a t-shirt when not at work.

During the interview, Lynn appeared thoughtful and pensive. She initially was cautious about self-disclosing, but as the interview proceeded, she became more open and candid in her responses. By the end of the interview, she was openly volunteering information about herself. She responded well to minor positive reinforcements and supportive comments. She indicated on a number of occasions that she appreciated feeling understood. Lynn appeared visibly anxious when discussing her future (both her vision of herself in relationships and her view of her work life), sad when discussing the death of her mother, and angry when discussing the end of her relationship. She expressed anger at the other driver when discussing the death of her father. Her speech ranged from slow and steady when discussing her mother to slightly rapid and pressured when discussing the loss of her relationship. Initially, Lynn was hesitant to make eye contact with the interviewer, but as the interview continued, she consistently did so.

She did not have difficulty expressing her feelings, and she appeared to appreciate having her feelings reflected back to her, as she stated that made her feel understood. Lynn's comments were consistently responsive to the questions asked and, as the interview proceeded, she was able to elaborate more fully.

Mood and Affect

Lynn reported feeling tense and pensive most days. She described herself as "jumpy" at work and said she felt anxious when people were physically close to her. She felt lethargic at home and anticipated that something else "bad" was going to happen to her. During the interview, Lynn's emotions were congruent with the content of the conversation, but underlying these emotions was a sense of dread, helplessness, and anxiety that things were not going to change. She rarely smiled or laughed. She did cry when discussing her mother's death and the breakup of her relationship. Overall, she appeared tense and on edge.

Thought Processes and Content/Orientation

Lynn was oriented to person, place, and time. Her short- and long-term memory appeared intact. She was alert, although she complained of being tired and of having difficulty falling asleep at night. She had a tendency to perseverate on her problems, and she reported difficulty concentrating and attending to details both at work and at home. Lynn's thought processes were intact and easy to follow and understand. She did not display delusions or hallucinations, although at one point she did say she thought she saw her mother walking in from her condo soon after she had died. Her judgment appeared good, and her intellectual ability was estimated to be above average.

Lynn did not express suicidal thoughts, and she explicitly stated that the cut on her hand was a cooking accident and she had no intention of hurting herself, nor had she ever harmed herself in any way. She also indicated that although she was still angry at her former partner, she had no intention to harm him. Her risk for violence to herself or others was assessed to be low.

Motivation for Treatment

Lynn's initial motivation for treatment as the session began was variable. She appeared to seek service in large part as an effort to appease her sister. As the interview continued and she felt supported and understood, her motivation for treatment increased. By the end of the interview, Lynn committed herself to working on the issues and concerns she discussed.

Assessment Considerations

Let us now turn our attention to considerations that will influence your assessment of Lynn. The first question to ask yourself with any patient is, What is the goal of the professional service you are offering? What is it that you are supposed to do, and what do you hope to accomplish? With Lynn, we knew that her behavior and emotions had changed recently and that she wanted to, as she said, "understand and change my behavior"—a statement that actually needs to be unpacked quite a lot.

First, there is not a specific referral question. Lynn was referred by her sister because her sister was concerned about her, but there is no directive to you about what you should do or what specific questions you are to address. Frequently, a referral is made for a psychological service with a specific goal in mind. That is particularly true when the psychological service is a formal assessment resulting in a written report, although such referrals are often made without a specific referral question, which is puzzling, as well as troubling. It seems intuitive to know that a question is more likely to be answered if the psychologist knows and understands exactly what the question is. When specific referral questions are not provided, referral sources need to be educated about how to make referrals. Sometimes there is also a referral question when the referral is for therapy. If the referral comes from a professional, that professional may have a particular goal in mind. If it comes from a family member or someone who knows the person well, that person may also have a particular goal in mind. For example, it is not infrequent in dealing with minors that the referral question is, in essence, "fix my kid," followed by a list of things that are "wrong" with the child or adolescent. However, it is also frequently the case that the referral is a self-referral, in which case there is no initial referral question, and one relies on the patient for identification of goals.

In this case, Lynn's goals have to do with understanding and changing her behavior, based on a growing sense of dread and decreased work productivity. We know from the psychological literature that understanding in and of itself is not what is most helpful in psychotherapy (Owen, Wong, & Rodolfa, 2010; Tracey, Lichtenberg, Goodyear, Claiborn, & Wampold, 2003), which raises the question, What is it that Lynn is really looking for? How does she conceptualize understanding her problems, and how does she think that enhancing her understanding will be helpful? How does she think about the path to that understanding and how, therefore, does she understand her current problems? Answering these and similar questions would require a fairly long discussion with her, with the initial goal to provide you with an understanding of what Lynn's thinking is and how she conceptualizes both herself and her perceived problems, as well as their solution.

Lynn is looking for behavior change. Although behavior change has been shown to be an effective means of improving one's life and feeling better about one's self and one's life (DeRubeis et al., 2005; Turner & Leach, 2012), that fact does not answer the question, Why is Lynn looking for behavior change? Does she have in mind specific behaviors she would like to change, or is it a more global change she desires? If she seeks specific changes, how and why did she choose those behaviors? What does she hope to accomplish by changing her behavior? In her thinking about herself and her life, what problems would behavior change solve and how? It is important to emphasize that these questions are not intended in any way as a challenge to her goal or her thinking regarding changing her life. Rather, they are intended to provide you with a better understanding of what her thinking and experiences are like. At this juncture, to stress the point, the goal of the discussion with Lynn is to gain a better understanding of her internal experience. A similar set of questions could be developed around the terms *dread* and *decreased work productivity.* We want to know early in the process of the assessment how Lynn sees herself and her life and what her style of reacting to herself and her life experiences is.

Let us take a step back from this case at this point and consider a bit the process we are now engaged in. One important message is that everything we do at the beginning of an assessment process revolves around understanding the person we are working with. What kind of a person is this? What are the person's life circumstances? Is his or her life challenging and difficult or relatively easy? What makes it difficult or easy? What kinds of external and internal resources does the person have? Given that, how does the person perceive him- or herself and the surrounding environment? Who are the important people in this person's life—or aren't there any? Is the person able to think logically and clearly about her life, or is she so overwhelmed that logic is simply not an option? Or is he a person who reacts emotionally and has difficulty thinking sequentially and logically? What impact do the person's cognitions seem to have on his or her life? What emotions are present, and how strong are they? How do they impact thoughts and behaviors?

As one can see, this a very long list of question to ask. However, doing a good assessment is not a matter of having all of the right questions in front of you and getting the person's answers. What is critical is understanding the internal experiences of the individual you are working with. That requires being focused on your patient and asking questions that grow out of what you are being told, rather than on a preconceived list of interview questions that appear on a sheet of paper in front of you. We have provided an interview outline in Appendix A that covers the topics we think will be important in doing a complete assessment. Many others are available, some of which we discuss in Chapter 9. We do not advocate simply going through an outline or a list of questions and getting information—perhaps information you think your supervisor might ask you about and you do not want to be embarrassed by saying you do not know. If that is a primary motivation, then the process is more about you than it is about your patient. We understand that early in training, it is inevitable that the process is in part about your learning, but eventually, the goal is to make the process about the patient, not about your needs. Doing a good assessment requires understanding the patient, learning about who that person is and how she experiences the world, as well as what resources and styles she has that you can use collaboratively to help her make the life changes desired. And to do that requires careful listening, but listening in a way different from social listening, where a primary goal of listening (if we are honest) is to look for opportunities to state our own opinions or talk about our own experiences. Listening in a professional relationship is of a very different quality. Carl Rogers, one of the fathers of clinical psychology, posed a series of questions that have to do with the nature of the professional relationship (C. R. Rogers, 1961, pp. 50–55). Every practicing psychologist, whether Rogerian in theoretical orientation or not, should read and think hard about such questions as, "Can I *be* in some way which will be perceived by the other person as trustworthy, as dependable or consistent in some deep sense" (p. 50) and "Can I let myself enter fully into the world of his [or her] feelings and personal meanings and see these as he [or she] does" (p. 53). The goal is listening closely enough to be able to ask ourselves, What does he mean by what was just said? What meaning or significance does that have for him? How does that relate to his internal experience and external behaviors? How does it relate to the work we have before us?

Diagnostic Considerations

The discussion above suggests that you still need to gather a considerable amount of information to understand Lynn's experience sufficiently for a competent assessment. Because you do not yet have all of that information, the following discussion on diagnostic considerations will of necessity be tentative. Our goal is not to provide the correct answer regarding her diagnosis but to lead you through the process that one should undertake to arrive at the most appropriate diagnosis.

A word here about this process. As we stated in Chapter 3, you will be gathering a great deal of information, from one or more of the five sources of data we discussed, depending on the nature and purpose of the assessment. The first step is to decide which of those data are most important. To make those decisions, you will need coursework that has taught you about normal and abnormal human behavior, that is, courses in personality, human development, cognition and affect, and psychopathology. Once you decide what is most important, you will need to compare those behaviors, cognitions, and emotions with what is in a diagnostic manual, such as the *Blue Book* or a textbook in psychopathology, to begin to formulate a list of possible, hypothetical, diagnostic categories that fit the signs and symptoms observed. Those diagnostic categories will then provide you with clues about other possible related symptoms that fit the diagnosis in question. Usually, especially early in your training, you will then need to go back to the patient and gather more information to determine whether the related symptoms are present. The final step, once you have determined, through multiple methods of data gathering, which signs and symptoms are present and are most crucial, is to compare those signs and symptoms with those most often present in your hypothetical diagnoses in order to ascertain the diagnosis that best fits the patient.

So, with regard to Lynn, what else might we need to know to develop an appropriate formulation and diagnosis? Let us start with the symptoms (meaning the problems as described by the patient) related to a potential diagnosis. What do we know? Most important, we know that Lynn is experiencing feelings of sadness and wants to stay home, finding it difficult to get out of the house and get to work. To stick with just these symptoms for a moment, what are the various possible (technically, called *differential*) diagnoses?[1]

Lynn could be experiencing depression, given her apparent lack of energy and interest in life. But, what kind of depression? She has had some major life stressors within the last few months: her mother's death and the end of a relationship. The impact of those events may be demonstrated in part by her level of physical activity. These contextual factors suggest that depression might be more episodic than ongoing. However, she is also experiencing physical symptoms related to her level of exercise. That information by itself might not be of immediate

---

[1]The less you know about a patient, the larger the list of potential diagnoses. The more information you have about the patient and the better your understanding of the ICD–10, the easier it will be to rule out some diagnoses and determine an appropriate one based on the patient's symptoms. This process of considering and ultimately eliminating possible diagnoses is called *differential diagnosis*.

concern, as it could indicate natural deconditioning, but it could also suggest the possibility of a physical ailment, or it could be a symptom of her depression. A psychologist should not attempt to think of differential diagnoses for medical illnesses, but a referral to a physician if symptoms are persistent or severe is certainly warranted.

What are Lynn's major symptoms, then, and which syndromes (diagnoses) do they best fit? At this point, consulting a diagnostic manual, the *Blue Book* for our purposes, is most helpful. The *Blue Book* lists what to look for when considering a diagnosis of depression (e.g., a change of mood or affect along with a change in activity, often related to a specific stressful event or situation; see p. 94), the specific symptoms one is likely to see ("depressed mood, loss of interest and enjoyment, and reduced energy leading to increased fatigability and diminished activity"; p. 100), and a list of other possible symptoms. The *Blue Book* also addresses the presence of anxiety in a primary diagnosis of depression, as well as the vegetative signs (e.g., sleep disturbance, psychomotor retardation, loss of appetite) one might see. It discusses which of the three varieties of depression— mild, moderate, and severe—is most appropriate, given the symptoms presented. The specific diagnostic guidelines regarding a depressive disorder state that, depending on whether the depression is mild, moderate, or severe, either two or three of the following symptoms should be present (pp. 101–102): depressed mood, loss of interest and enjoyment, and increased fatigability, plus two to four or more of the other symptoms listed (reduced concentration and attention, reduced self-esteem and self-confidence, ideas of guilt and worthlessness, bleak and pessimistic views of the future, ideas or acts of self-harm or suicide, disturbed sleep, diminished appetite; p. 100). Thus, the *Blue Book* provides a fair amount of guidance regarding which symptoms to look for and the types of symptom configurations that are usually present in each of the specific diagnoses. Note that we said "usually": The ICD–10 (WHO, 2016) system provides the clinician with a certain amount of judgment to determine which diagnosis or diagnoses best fit the clinical picture. Whenever you have questions regarding a specific diagnosis, we recommend you consult a diagnostic manual.

What, then, are the various signs and symptoms in Lynn's presentation? The following key experiences can be noted: feels a sense of dread and helplessness; work productivity has suffered; drags self to work; experiences anxiety, tension, fatigue, lethargy, and anger; has concentration difficulties; has decreased physical activity; and uses alcohol. With these general guidelines and list of signs and symptoms in mind, one can see that Lynn's presentation certainly fits a depressive disorder, specifically a major depressive disorder, although she is able to get to work and there is not evidence at this point of psychotic features (intact thought processes, lack of hallucinations or delusions, good judgment, general orientation, and adequate memory, although seeing her mother walking into the room after her death should be explored). If there were psychotic features, the ICD–10–CM code would be F32.3. The current symptoms seem more suggestive of Major depressive disorder, single episode of either a moderate (F32.1) or severe (F32.2) nature, with all three of the primary symptoms being present and at least three of the other listed symptoms. (It also is highly likely, given her presentation, that lowered self-esteem and, possibly, feelings of guilt or worthlessness are present, so those possibilities should be further explored with her.) If depression, the possibility of Suicidal ideations (R45.851) should be considered, especially in light of the bandage she had on her hand, which could be an indication of self-harm (Intentional self-harm by knife [F78.1]), in spite of her claims that it was an accident.

On the other hand, this constellation of symptoms could be an anxiety disorder, given her general emotional discomfort and your observations during the interview. Checking the *Blue Book* for symptoms of anxiety, the following are relevant: presentation with anxiety and tension and difficulty concentrating. Such behavioral observations are an important source of psychological data. Again, though, there are multiple possibilities. Lynn might have an anxiety disorder, specifically, Generalized anxiety disorder (F41.1), or she might be reacting more to particularly stressful environmental events, of short duration (symptoms began within 1 month of a stressful event and have not been present for more than 6 months), resulting in an adjustment disorder. An adjustment disorder has a range of options: It could be an adjustment disorder with no greater specification because no particular symptom stands out as determinative (Adjustment disorder, unspecified [F43.20]), it could be an adjustment disorder that presents with depression as the primary symptom (Adjustment disorder with depressed mood [F43.21]), or with anxiety as the primary symptom (F43.22), or with mixed anxiety and depressed mood (F43.23). When one looks further at the ICD–10–CM, one sees even more possibilities, with conduct being the primary disturbance (F43.24), or with mixed disturbance in both conduct and emotion (F43.25) or, even, a category that does not fit any of those specific presentations, Adjustment disorder with other symptoms (F43.29).

A variety of other possible diagnoses, such as a Persistent mood disorder (F34.x), Major depressive disorder, recurrent (F33.x), or Obsessive-compulsive disorder (F42; reflecting her perseveration) are possibilities, but you would need more evidence for such diagnoses. More information is obviously needed. Given her current use of alcohol, Alcohol abuse (F10.1x) is also a consideration. Although alcohol use does not seem to be the primary problem, it often complicates, and sometimes makes impossible, progress in psychotherapy (Hester

& Miller, 2002). As a result, it is important to consider Lynn's alcohol intake carefully.

As stated above but worth repeating, we currently have no firm basis for making a differential diagnosis that best fits Lynn's symptoms. All of our diagnostic statements to this point should be considered as hypotheses that need to be ruled out. What we are doing is considering all of the possible diagnostic categories on the basis of the data we currently have. This process should lead us to think of the appropriate questions that would provide answers necessary to understand the person and to determine the best diagnosis. The fine distinctions these diagnoses (or others not yet considered here) provide might be crucial to the question of what is the best way to move forward, meaning in Lynn's case, what kinds of therapeutic interventions would likely be most helpful.

As you can see, thinking carefully about the diagnosis helps us to consider what the patient's individual and specific experiences are like. Stated another way, we believe that a thorough consideration of the differential diagnoses leads to a more complete and accurate conceptualization of the person. That is, a consideration of the possible diagnostic categories helps us develop the important questions that will lead us to better understand the patient. And understanding the patient is crucial to developing an intervention approach that will most likely help Lynn achieve her goals.

In Lynn's case, therefore, we need to know the answer to questions such as, How severe is her emotional disturbance? How pervasive is it in her life and to what degree does it affect her ability to function, her relationships, and her subjective sense of satisfaction in her life? Is it always present or does it come and go? How long has she felt this way, and was its onset something fairly sudden (more likely, then, to be a reaction to some external event), or has it actually been coming on for a long time? Or was an underlying emotional disturbance always present, and it was just her immediate emotional state that was precipitated by life events (possibly indicating a gradually developing reaction to chronic stressors in her life or a stronger genetic component, less triggered by her environment)? The answers to those specific types of questions and following up whatever threads her answers provide will help us differentiate between chronic and episodic dysfunction, as well as mild, moderate, and severe disorders.

The various possibilities under the Adjustment disorders category would lead us to ask questions about the exact nature of Lynn's emotional reactions, from her subjective experience. How does she experience her emotional reactions, and are they constant or changing? Do her problems express themselves primarily in behavioral terms, or is there a combination of emotional discomfort and disturbed or disturbing behavior? Do her emotions seem to her to tend toward the constellation of depressive or anxiety symptoms?

We also know that she has difficulty with concentration and focus. Does that provide us any diagnostic help? Probably not by itself. Both depression and anxiety can result in difficulties with concentration and focus, although for different reasons. Certainly, exploring with her the nature of those difficulties could be enlightening, both diagnostically and in understanding what Lynn's experience is like.

A number of other factors are important to consider in trying to understand Lynn and determine the types of interventions that would be most helpful. Lynn lives alone. At this point, we do not know what that means. It could be a positive indication of independence. It could mean that she is lonely, because she is naturally a gregarious person and living alone does not provide her sufficient interpersonal interaction. It could mean that she is lonely because she has lived with other people her entire life and only recently started living alone. If the latter, was that by her choice, or was that decision made for her, such as in the breakup of her relationship? Besides the external variables associated with living alone, how does she experience it? Is it enjoyable for her or undesirable? Does she look forward to being home alone or dread it, or something in between? How did it happen that she started living alone, and how long ago did that happen? The important point we are making is that you should not make assumptions about what a seemingly simple fact means for a patient. You cannot know what it means for her unless you ask her about it.

Living alone is a very good example of a situation that we all have some reaction to, either because we now live alone, we have lived alone, or we have avoided or sought living alone. Precisely because it is such a common human experience, it is also extremely important that we not let our own feelings and reactions to the idea of living alone influence how we approach the issue with Lynn. We cannot and must not assume that her experience will be at all like ours is or has been. It is very important that we allow her to have her own experience, that we not read our experience into hers, but that we listen carefully and with empathy to how she experiences living alone. Remember, as her psychologist, your goal is to understand her experience.

It is also important to maintain some degree of objectivity. That means that you must avoid getting drawn too intimately into the patient's story. One can understand and empathize with, without being drawn into, the life experience being described. How one reacts to a person who is describing difficult experiences is also important. You should not overstate the amount of understanding you have of the experiences being described. The more heart-wrenching those experiences are, the less likely you are really to understand, even if you have had similar experiences, as each experience is unique and each individual is unique. Thus, be cautious of saying you understand, for it creates the risk of appearing simply shallow and superficial. The risk is that the people you are listening to might well say in their own heads, "You can't possibly understand what this was like for me," or question, "How can you possibly understand, you are too (young, old, male, female) different from me?" When that happens, the relationship experiences a rupture that may be difficult to repair.

We do know that family is involved in Lynn's case. She has a positive relationship with her sister, although exactly how close they are and how much of a support her sister is, we do not know yet, except that her sister lives at some geographic distance. Lynn appeared to have a special relationship with her mother. Her father was tragically killed when she was 6, so her mother may have taken on an especially important role for her. That can have numerous repercussions and meanings, which should be explored. Her mother's death was likely a major event for her and might have been a major contributing factor to her current psychological problems. The quantity and quality of psychological resources Lynn has, including interpersonal support, may be central to determining whether the psychological problems she is having are of a mild, moderate, or severe nature.

Lynn's loss of a romantic relationship within the past 5 months adds another layer of emotional stress and may have primary implications for the supports available to her and the resources she has to work with. The way in which the relationship ended might also have had an impact on how she feels about herself and the level of trust she believes she can have in other people, perhaps meaning that her psychological and interpersonal resources are even more limited. The possibility that she is grieving the loss of social supports might provide useful data about whether her emotional disturbance is more depression or anxiety. Some people react to loss by feeling profoundly sad; others, by feeling extremely anxious about how they will manage without the support they had. In addition, people may react with anger, which is not considered a diagnostic disorder unless it reflects a personality style, such as Antisocial personality disorder (F60.2), or fits an R code in the ICD–10–CM (i.e., signs and symptoms that do not have specific diagnoses), such as Irritability and anger (R45.4), Hostility (R.45.5), Violent behavior (R45.6), or anger without Homicidal ideation (R45.850). Certainly people can be angry at partners who betray them, but they can also be angry at loved ones who die and leave them.

Lynn does still have some social supports in the form of friends who live close to her and who check in with her. However, the degree to which she is able to experience that support, given her possible irritability about their suggestions about her seeking help, is not clear. That is also an issue worth exploring with her.

The bit of data about Lynn's reaction to her friends also has potential implications for her involvement in therapy. If that is the reaction she had, does that mean that she is involved in therapy with reluctance, despite her supposed commitment? Against her better wishes? Was she indeed in therapy primarily to "appease her sister?" Might she carry some animosity from her friends toward you? Will she be resistant to any input or suggestions made by you for those reasons? Does she carry negative feelings about psychotherapy generally, given that she does not believe the therapy she received after her father died was helpful? This is a good example of one small bit of information that can have wide-ranging implications. It means that it is crucial for you to be thinking beyond the information of what is being said to the meaning or importance of that information for the patient's life.

We also know that Lynn's work performance is an issue. Her worry about job security suggests anxiety, but these kinds of stressors can also result in feelings of being overwhelmed and depressed, which are prime issues for exploration with Lynn.

In addition to this myriad of specific questions in Lynn's case, some basic questions should be a part of every assessment, whether formal, with written report, or informal. What are the person's general strengths? What does this person do well? Where has this person had success in her life? In what ways does she feel good about herself and her life? Beyond general strengths, what are the specific strengths/skills that allow her to manage in her life? Every person copes to some degree with stressors, even when generally the person feels overwhelmed. What, specifically, does she do that enables her to live her life with whatever level of productivity, personal satisfaction and comfort, and interpersonal warmth exists? When hard times or challenging situations come, what works to lessen the load or overcome the troubles?

A second major area of inquiry should concern the vulnerabilities the person has. What experiences or situations cause him or her the most pain? Where are the person's weaknesses? What are the behaviors or reactions that seem to work least well in coping with difficult circumstances? Where does the person feel most inadequate and most overwhelmed?

Although the first two general categories focus on the individual himself/herself, the last one focuses on the environment. What are the triggers in this person's life? What sets her off? What makes her feel particularly inadequate and vulnerable? What has she attempted to do in the past to cope with these situations and how do they defeat her despite her best efforts?

Closing Comments

If the assessment is intended to answer specific referral questions, a discussion of the person's strengths, weaknesses, and triggers may provide the core of what can be said. If the purpose of the assessment is an attempt to help the person cope more effectively, some additional questions regarding the relationship between the three categories might be helpful, such as, Can this person's strengths be used in a different, more effective manner to help cope better, or are new coping skills likely to be necessary? What can be done to minimize the weaknesses that exist? Can the strengths be strengthened in a way that will work or, are new skills necessary to overcome the weaknesses that are present? How has the person conceptualized the trigger situations in her life? Have the responses been inadequate or, in some way, misplaced? In other words, are new skills or behaviors required or can more effective use of current skills suffice?

What does all of this mean for the ultimate ICD–10–CM diagnosis? As we have stated, we do not yet know what that ought to be, because we need additional data to answer that question. At this point, your diagnostic thinking should include Lynn's overall presentation and additional data you collect, which may answer your question about whether she is more depressed or anxious. Thus, it seems that the most likely central differential diagnoses are Major depressive disorder, single episode, moderate (F32.1); Generalized anxiety disorder (F41.1); or Adjustment disorder with depressed mood (F43.21), or with anxiety as the primary symptom (F43.22). Narrowing down the potential diagnoses helps you focus on the questions that are most important for you to understand Lynn's experiences.

Using the ICD–10–CM

Case 2—John Smith

5

A 47-year-old African American man named John Smith is referred to you for an assessment by his cardiologist, Dr. Jones, to identify underlying psychological issues and for possible follow-up for psychological treatment. She would like a full, formal assessment to ensure completeness, but no other information is provided in the referral letter. The exact language in the letter states, "Please conduct a complete assessment to determine psychological diagnosis and possible disposition and provide a report in two weeks. Thank you." You note in your own mind that you have received numerous referrals from Dr. Jones in the past without a great deal of specificity. You have taken seriously the notion to train your referral sources to ask more specific questions, but you have been unsuccessful with Dr. Jones, as she has indicated in the past that she sometimes is too busy to provide patient information in the referral, as you can find the information in the patient's chart. You contact her office and are told that she is out of town at a conference and will not be back for a week.

http://dx.doi.org/10.1037/14778-006
A Student's Guide to Assessment and Diagnosis Using the ICD–10–CM: Psychological and Behavioral Conditions, by J. Schaffer and E. Rodolfa

It is even possible that Dr. Jones's nurse drafted the letter. You call the cardiologist's office to talk with the nurse practitioner, and sure enough, she does not know exactly what Dr. Jones would like to know. So, as sometimes is the case, you will need to make the best of the limited information that you have. You could, on the basis of that limited (inadequate) information, decline the referral, but if you work in a medical setting and react that way, you will probably have a difficult time getting enough referrals to earn a living.

What might you do to make the best of this situation? You do know that your prospective evaluee is hospitalized. Therefore, the first step might be to go to the hospital and read through his chart, which might provide you not only with useful psychological information but also some medical history that will likely be helpful to know, given that the primary diagnosis of this person has to do with his heart.

You find out from your review of Mr. Smith's chart that his diagnosis according to the Clinical Modification of the *International Statistical Classification of Diseases and Related Health Problems* (ICD–10–CM; National Center for Health Statistics, 2015) is Unstable angina (I20.0). You have worked with cardiac patients in the past. In fact, you did a rotation during your postdoctoral training year in an inpatient cardiology unit. But you have not worked with a patient with this specific diagnosis yet. That raises a question of limits of competence, which we discuss in Chapter 7, this volume.

You further discover that Mr. Smith is a chemist who works in the research section of a local large company that, among other products, manufactures antifungal agents for use in agriculture. The medical chart indicates that Mr. Smith experiences considerable job-related stress, although the exact nature of the stress is not clear. You are also surprised to learn that the company he works for is the same company your significant other's brother works for.

The chart provides some personal history. Mr. Smith grew up in a rural area of the country, the son of a high school chemistry teacher. He attended the state university in his home state and then went to California Institute of Technology (Cal Tech) for graduate school. He is married and has three children living at home.

Medically, he began having chest pain for the first time 2 months ago. Prior to that time, he had not experienced any symptoms and, in fact, had felt quite healthy, although his doctor told him that his blood sugars were borderline. He put off seeing his physician, because he thought the pain he was having was either indigestion or a result of stress-related anxiety, until the pain became fairly severe 2 days before his hospitalization. At that time, he called his primary care physician's office and, on the basis of the nature and severity of the symptoms, they called 911 and had Mr. Smith taken to the emergency department of the local hospital. He was then admitted to the cardiology unit. He is slightly overweight, had nonfasting blood sugars of 120, heart rate of 85, blood pressure of 150/90, but he is otherwise healthy.

The chart provides little other information that is relevant to your assessment. It provides you with no indication of the specific questions the cardiologist might have.

Assessment Considerations

Given this limited information, what is it that we know about Mr. Smith, and what clinical issues or questions are raised? The first issue is that this is, obviously, a very different type of referral from that discussed in Chapter 4. It is not a referral for psychotherapy (at least not initially), but specifically for an assessment. We very purposely included such a case because, although not every psychologist engages in formal psychological testing, testing and psychological assessment is one of the services psychologists offer that is unique to our profession.

Very little information was provided with the referral letter, leaving you at a decided disadvantaged (as we discussed in Chapter 3). It is difficult to answer questions completely and accurately when one does not know what the questions are.

The first step is to seek as much background information as possible, although in some cases, such as this one, it might be difficult to determine exactly why a referral is being made. When that is the situation, one does the best that one can. That includes, in particular, developing one's own set of referral questions, that is, your developing sense of what needs to be addressed as you collect data about the potential reasons someone has been referred for a psychological assessment. The best source of such information would be the patient himself or herself. In this case, you would gradually, through a variety of data sources, begin to develop a sense of who Mr. Smith is, what his concerns or questions or fears are, and the impact those issues have on his life. From there, developing a set of implied referral questions is often not so complex a process.

A good starting point in a health psychology context is with the medical diagnosis. The more one knows about the medical aspects of the person's problems, the more conversant one can be with the language medical professionals use, and the more one is likely to have some understanding of what the subjective experience of the patient might be. Hence, consulting with a decent general text in internal medicine that includes a review of cardiology might be beneficial (see, e.g., Wiener, Fauci, Braunwald, Kasper, & Hauser, 2012). Working in a medical setting does not require that one become knowledgeable at the level of a physician or a nurse, but if the psychologist does not have curiosity about the kinds of issues medical professionals face and the kinds of experiences medical patients have, working in such a setting is probably not a good fit.

In this case, as in many situations, start with a review of the available data, especially the patient's chart. Without knowing the referral questions, it is difficult to know what exactly one should be looking for. A medical chart would be full of medical test data (e.g., lab values, EKG, echocardiogram), as well as nursing notes that have to do with vital signs (temperature, blood pressure, heart rate, respiration rate), eating schedule, and so on. Much of that is not particularly relevant for a psychologist, but sometimes it contains information that is relevant to the particular concerns of the patient. In particular, nursing notes are often a rich source of information about the day-to-day functioning and psychological conditions of medical inpatients. So, at least scanning the nursing notes is recommended. One might also hope (and expect) that the progress notes of the physician or physicians would contain information about why a referral to a psychologist was considered. A conversation with the charge nurse on the unit or with the nurse who has provided the most care for Mr. Smith might also be helpful, but confidentiality considerations play an important role, which we examine more fully in Chapter 7.

There is another issue to consider before we start a discussion of the process of undertaking an assessment. Your significant other's brother (let's call him Mark) works in the same company as Mr. Smith. That raises an ethical consideration that we consider in more detail in Chapter 7. At this point, if you believe there is no conflict of interest or other reason for you to reject the referral, the next step would be a conversation with Mr. Smith about whether he thinks this presents a prohibitive conflict of interest. In a hospital setting, it is helpful to check with the nursing staff first to see what the patient's schedule might be, to be sure he is available.

In addition, when working in an outpatient setting, it is reasonable to assume that a person coming to see you does so voluntarily and with certain goals (or, at least, thoughts on what might be helpful about the process). You cannot necessarily assume that in an inpatient setting. So, the first task is a discussion with Mr. Smith about whether he wants to see you. Such a conversation might provide a great deal of information about Mr. Smith's current situation, emotional state, and goals. Or it might not. It might take more questioning and discussion to find out what Mr. Smith's views and goals are. Whichever way the discussion goes, however, you have collected useful information about Mr. Smith. You know that he is either a willing and enthusiastic participant in an assessment process or he is reluctant, closed, cautious, or suspicious or downright resistant. Now, in addition to the information you have on his medical condition and something of his work situation and its potential relationship to his angina, you have information about how he relates to you, to Dr. Jones, and to the referral. That opens three potential avenues (his medical status, his work status, and his interactive ability) for discussion with Mr. Smith. Which of those three paths you take depends on a number of factors and is beyond the scope of this text. Most readers will have had coursework in interviewing before reading this book or will have such coursework soon. If not, check Chapter 10, this volume, for possible resources in the area to consult, remembering that in addition to consulting the psychological literature, both in the form of journal articles and books, one needs to receive supervision in the provision of virtually any psychological service from a competent supervisor to be adept at providing that psychological service.

Let us now flesh out the data we have available to decide how best to proceed with the assessment process and with the conclusions regarding diagnosis and ultimate disposition. In Mr. Smith's case, you have been responsible for seeking out the information, as very little of it was forthcoming easily. So, let us assume the following information, based on your review of the medical chart, your interview with Mr. Smith, and possibly, collateral interviews (e.g., with Mr. Smith's family members, work colleagues, work supervisors). (Collateral interviews are discussed further in Chapter 7.)

So, who is Mr. Smith? He tells you about growing up in the rural South, the third of four children of a high school chemistry teacher and a stay-at-home mother. The family was quite close, although all of the children felt the high expectations placed on them by their parents. Grandparents on both sides had been lower middle-class farmers, so his father had worked very hard to put himself through college to become a teacher. Mr. Smith had always felt the pressure of living up to his father's expectation and has generally been successful in doing so, graduating with honors from his state university and receiving a masters' degree from Cal Tech, although he always feared that his acceptance and success there was in part a function of affirmative action rather than his abilities, a notion he reacts to with some irritability.

Mr. Smith is in a committed gay relationship, and he and his partner have three adopted children, ages 8, 10, and 17. If you assumed up to this point that married with children meant a heterosexual relationship with biological children, consider what that says about your biases. His partner works as a police officer. Together, their income is well within the middle class, but they have very high expectations for their three children and the cost of private schools is very high, so they are feeling some financial stress. Both he and his partner experience some discrimination, both because of their sexual orientation and their ethnic backgrounds. In addition, although his partner's job is not a 9-to-5 job, he is frequently called in for emergencies. They have had some struggles about work hours and finding someone to be responsible for the two younger children without relying too much on the 17-year-old, which has resulted in some difficult interactions between him and his partner and between the two of them and their oldest child.

Mr. Smith has been very successful working for All Chemical Company; he has worked there for 6 years, following two previous positions in a different city. He has a good working relationship with his boss, although he tends to feel inferior to him, who is a doctorally trained chemist and whom Mr. Smith views as a genius. Mr. Smith has been working on a new chemical and is feeling a great deal of pressure because his boss believes that a rival company is working on a similar, though not identical, chemical. His boss believes that the company that brings its product to the market first is likely to have a significant advantage in market share. Mr. Smith has always worked very long hours, believing that he had to be better than most to be considered their equal. Recently, he has felt that even longer hours are required, so he typically leaves their home before 7:00 a.m. and is usually not home until around 9:00 p.m.

Mr. Smith presented as very interactive, responsive, and cooperative with the interview process. He appeared to be very bright, on more than one occasion answering the question before you completed it—and doing so correctly, that is, he was able to correctly understand the intent of your question before you finished asking it. That style also revealed to you a certain degree of impatience. He talked more rapidly than the average person and seemed jittery. As he discussed his work situation in particular, it was evident that he feels considerable stress, but sometimes both his financial condition and his social interactions are also difficult for him. Last, Mr. Smith is obviously concerned about his health. He does not know at this point what implications for lifestyle and workload his heart disease will have, and that is worrisome for him.

From the interview, what do you now know about Mr. Smith? You know about his supportive family with high standards, to which Mr. Smith has reacted with some underlying feelings of inadequacy. His current family life is also supportive and, from Mr. Smith's perspective, very successful but not without its stresses, as well. He is very successful professionally, in large part as a result of his competence but also because of his work ethic. His general intellectual and interpersonal competence means that he is able to deal with most situations in his life very effectively, although his underlying feelings of inadequacy are a challenge for him. He denies use of alcohol or drugs, which is supported by the level of productivity he demonstrates in a job that is intellectually challenging.

Given this set of facts, what additional data would you want? Mr. Smith has not obtained psychological services in the past, so there are no psychological records to seek. You have had access to the medical records. Other records, such as educational records, are unlikely to add much to this clinical picture and have the additional problems of confidentiality and logistics in obtaining them. Likewise, there is no reason to believe, given the information that you have, that collateral interviews would add much useful information.

That leaves psychological test data, which can be obtained without great difficulty. What testing data might you want? A large number of questions do not need to be answered, so a large battery of tests probably is neither necessary nor worth the cost. Given his presentation during the interview and his level of vocational success, it is unlikely that taking the time to administer a general test of intelligence would be worthwhile and provide useful information to the cardiologist. You would likely find out what you have already concluded. Mr. Smith is considerably brighter than average. No major psychological disorders are present, although it might be helpful to get confirmation of that hypothesis from psychological test data. So, we would probably want to get a general test of psychological disorders, such as the Minnesota Multiphasic Personality Inventory—2 (MMPI–2) or the Personality Assessment Inventory (PAI; Morey, 1991). Nothing indicates an underlying personality disorder, which is helpful because no tests are available that provide reliable and valid diagnostic impressions for personality disorders. However, especially in a person without major psychological dysfunction, a measure of normal personality function, such as the NEO Personality Inventory–III (NEO-PI-III; Costa & McCrae, 2005), the California Personality Inventory—Revised (CPI–R; Gough, 1987), or the 16-PF might be instructive. A projective test like the Thematic Apperception Test (TAT; Murray, 1943) or the Rorschach (Rorschach, 1927) might also provide useful personality information, although you would need to ask yourself whether the time required for administration and scoring would provide sufficient reliable information, in addition to what you already know or the other tests will provide you, to be worth the expense involved in gathering such information (see, e.g., Wood, Nezworski, Lilienfeld, & Garb, 2003).

Given the set of circumstances described in this case, we would likely start with the MMPI–2, as it provides a fairly broad-based test of psychological dysfunction. It could provide value just in case something important was missed in the file review and interview that indicates a psychological disorder is in fact present. The PAI is somewhat more closely aligned with current taxonomies, such as the ICD–10 and the *Diagnostic and Statistical Manual of Mental Disorders, Fifth Edition* (American Psychiatric Association, 2013), but in the absence of any clear diagnostic hypothesis, the breadth of the MMPI–2 might cover more ground. In this case, the shorter Minnesota Multiphasic Personality Inventory—Restructured Clinical (MMPI–RC; Tellegen et al., 2003) is also an option.

On the other hand, our experience is that the MMPI–2 or MMPI–RC and the PAI often provide slightly different information. Given that little expense is involved in either test, if Mr. Smith is cooperative and willing to take both tests, it might make sense to administer both to him.

Last, we would administer a test of normal personality to obtain a better sense than tests of pathology provide on the coping styles a person uses. In addition, in our experience the two types of tests often are somewhat mutually exclusive, in the sense that the test of normal personality often adds little helpful information when a great deal of pathology is present (i.e., when there is considerable elevation on the profiles of the MMPI–2 and/or the PAI). Conversely, when relatively little pathology is present, such that the MMPI–2 or the PAI have little, if any, elevation and provide limited data, the test of normal personality can be extremely rich in information. One author of this text, although trained in the use of the CPI–R, began to use the NEO-PI-R because it reflects the mostly widely accepted and researched model of personality, the five-factor model (McCrae & Costa, 1987; Wiggins, 1996) and found the test extremely beneficial.

Diagnostic Considerations

In this situation, we encourage you to go through the same process of hypothesis generation, data collection, and decision making as we did in the case described in Chapter 4. Now we consider the information we have and need to make a diagnosis.

Without the benefit of the psychological test data, but assuming accuracy of the information we have gathered during the clinical interview, what implications do the data we have acquired have in determining an ICD–10–CM diagnosis—and what implications do the diagnostic considerations have for the kinds of data you might look for in the psychological tests? First, on the basis of medical data, you know that Mr. Smith has a diagnosis of Unstable angina (I20.0). What are the psychological symptoms that seem to be most important? You know that he is under considerable stress—job, financial, and family related—and feels burdened by that stress. He also appears to have feelings of inadequacy and inferiority. He reports being worried about his health. He presents as somewhat jittery, mildly hyperactive, and mildly impatient. Although it would be natural for such a person to feel some depression, and ruling out depression is one purpose of giving a test like the MMPI–2 or the PAI, Mr. Smith appears to present more with anxiety than depression. His anxiety does not appear to be debilitating, as he has been able to cope reasonably well and continues to be productive at work. At the same time, it may well be that his anxiety is a contributing factor to his vascular occlusions, although you cannot know whether the relationship is causal. You do know (or would learn through reading and experience if you are competent to take on a referral such as this) that psychological distress is a significant risk factor for heart disease (Smith & Ruiz, 2002; Stansfeld, Fuhrer, Shipley, & Marmot, 2002).

No evidence indicates, and you have no reason to speculate, that cognitive dysfunction is related to cardiac insufficiency (Vascular dementia; F01.50), but you might keep this tucked in the back of your mind as a future possibility (Battistin & Cagnin, 2010). You know that he is concerned about his health, so a diagnosis of a Mood disorder due to known physiological condition (F06.3; here, a blockage of one or more coronary arteries) is a possibility, although Anxiety disorder due to known physiological condition (F06.4) may be more likely, given his presentation. Nothing indicates Alcohol abuse (F10.1) or Alcohol dependency (F10.2), and Mr. Smith denies they are relevant, although given the prevalence of self-medication using alcohol or drugs in individuals with depression or anxiety, those diagnoses should always be considered.

Thus far, you have a medical diagnosis of Unstable angina (I20.0) and a possible mental health diagnosis of Anxiety disorder due to known physiological condition (F06.4), although the latter appears to be a secondary diagnosis, as the primary emotional distress comes not from his medical condition, but from his work and, somewhat less so, from his social life. Therefore, a number of diagnostic categories are possibilities as the primary psychological diagnosis, given the symptoms described. Mr. Smith could have Generalized anxiety disorder (F41.1), given indications of lack of self-confidence and emotional distress since childhood, along with apprehension and motor tension, symptoms listed in the *Blue Book* (World Health Organization, 1993, p. 116). Or, some degree of depression may be present, which additional interviewing or the testing data might reveal and which could result in a diagnosis of Mixed anxiety and depressive disorder (F41.2) or, even, an Other mixed anxiety disorder (F41.3), depending on whether other anxiety-related symptoms are discovered through additional interviewing or testing, or an Anxiety disorder, unspecified (F41.9). Given his general level of productivity and emotional stability, however, it might be that his current distress is primarily a result of the stressors he is experiencing in his life. The degree of stress does not appear to be sufficient to warrant a diagnosis of Acute stress reaction (F43.0) or Posttraumatic stress disorder (F43.1), given that the level of stress in those disorders is usually of an overwhelming degree, such as threat to life or psychological integrity.

Mr. Smith could well be experiencing an Adjustment disorder (F43.2), however, which can result from a "period of adaptation to the consequences of a stressful life event (including the presence or possibility of serious physical illness)" (*Blue Book*, p. 121). In the case of an adjustment disorder, the general considerations we discussed above, strengths, weaknesses, and triggers, will be particularly crucial, given the *Blue Book* statement:

> Individual predisposition or vulnerability plays a greater role in the risk of occurrence and shaping of the manifestations of adjustment disorders than it does in the other conditions in F43.–, but it is nevertheless assumed that the condition would not have arisen without the stressor. (p. 121)

The *Blue Book* makes a similar point about the importance of considering broader issues in stating, "Diagnosis depends on a careful evaluation of the relationship between (a) form, content, and severity of symptoms; (b) previous history and personality; and (c) stressful event, situation, or life crisis" (p. 121). Psychological testing data might be particularly useful in providing such broader perspectives.

Although multiple questions are to be answered before a final diagnosis can be reached, given the data we have, our primary psychological working diagnosis would be Generalized anxiety disorder (F41.1), given Mr. Smith's current level of anxiety and long-standing issues with self-esteem and emotional distress. At this point in the process, one should think about a working diagnosis as a starting point, from which questions arise, the answers to which lead to the final diagnosis. So given what you know, do you agree with our working diagnosis or do you have other potential diagnoses that you are considering?

Closing Comments

This chapter has provided you with numerous questions that would potentially be explored in a thorough assessment of this patient. Once that thorough assessment is completed, you will be able to formulate a final diagnosis. This chapter also highlighted a number of issues regarding consultation and referral, in addition to the process of assessment and diagnosis. Regardless of the location of your practice, whether it is an independent practice or in an integrated health center, it is critical for you to develop positive working relationships and an ability to professionally consult with your colleagues from other professions.

Using the ICD–10–CM
Case 3—Anne Sanchez

6

Y ou recently began your practice in a small city after having been licensed as a psychologist 3 years ago. After working in a hospital in a much larger city, you and your life partner decided that you wanted to move to a smaller town with a slower pace of life. You appreciate the relationships you have already been able to build with members of the health care community, and you have hospital privileges at the closest hospital, which is about 20 minutes away from your office. You are one of three psychologists in town and the three of you are on good terms, are helpful to one another, and consult regularly with each other.

You receive a referral from an attorney who works at a resource center for indigent and homeless individuals. The attorney refers Anne Sanchez, a 36-year-old, single, Mexican American woman. Ms. Sanchez was homeless for several years and recently has been living in her mother's converted garage in your town. An evaluation was requested to determine specifically if Ms. Sanchez has a mental disability

http://dx.doi.org/10.1037/14778-007
A Student's Guide to Assessment and Diagnosis Using the ICD–10–CM: Psychological and Behavioral Conditions, by J. Schaffer and E. Rodolfa

resulting in functional impairment, which might qualify her for federal supplemental income programs. Ms. Sanchez is bilingual, fluent in English and Spanish, having grown up in a family that primarily spoke Spanish but attended a school where English was used.

Ms. Sanchez's presenting complaints were constant sadness, difficulty concentrating, and poor ability to report facts accurately. She complained of physical problems, including fatigue and pain in her legs, arms, and hands. She also reported that voices tell her to harm herself by running onto the freeway. She stated that when the voices become persistent, she takes at least two and sometimes more sleeping pills to fall asleep as a way of coping, because she also has a strong desire to live.

Ms. Sanchez has an extended history of polysubstance abuse (cocaine, alcohol). However, she stated that she has not used alcohol or cocaine for more than 2 years, which was corroborated by her physician, Dr. Winters. Ms. Sanchez explained that about 2.5 years ago, she went to a substance abuse treatment program and feels committed to using the techniques and incorporating the attitudes she learned there. Currently, she reported feeling stress due to her living situation and lack of energy that impairs her functioning. She described having few friends and does not trust others, because of past experiences of being harmed by people with whom she had close relationships. Ms. Sanchez reported sleeping most afternoons as a way to pass time and cope with her bad moods. She expressed suicidal ideation but did not have intent or a plan and described a strong will to live and to attempt to reunite with her children.

Ms. Sanchez was often uncertain about exact dates or years when events actually occurred. She was born in a neighboring town approximately 100 miles away from where she now lives. She has never traveled far out of the local area. Ms. Sanchez is the middle child, initially with two brothers and two sisters. One brother died in a car accident when Ms. Sanchez was 12 years old, and a sister was found dead in her own apartment about a year ago. There was speculation of a purposeful drug overdose, but there was no note, and her sister's death was ruled an accidental drug overdose.

Ms. Sanchez has a son (age 14) and a daughter (age 18). She lost custody of her children 12 years ago because of drug and alcohol problems; at that time, she went to jail for possession of cocaine.

Her father, an electrician, died of a heart attack when she was 16 years old. She recounted tearfully that his death was very difficult for her. Ms. Sanchez described her mother as distant, uninvolved, and having difficulty providing for the family once her father died. She reported that she turned to prostitution after her father's death as a way of providing income for her family, sometimes with men as the customer and sometimes, women. It was, simply, a source of badly needed income for her and her family. She left high school at the start of her senior year to take care of her first child. She was uncertain about the identity of the father of her child. She estimated that she started drinking heavily in her teens after her father died and started using drugs in her 20s. She reported being sexually molested as a teenager by relatives, including an uncle and a female family friend. She described a suicide attempt, "taking a lot of pills," but she was vague about when that happened (either in her late 20s or early 30s) and was vague in describing what she wanted to have happen.

In her early 20s, Ms. Sanchez received her GED, which allowed her to enter community college and also to attend cosmetology school. However, she did not finish her community college degree and completed only three classes at cosmetology school. Previous employment included working in a beauty shop washing hair and scheduling appointments, working at a preschool as a child care worker, and most recently as a telemarketer. She reported not being employed during the past year. She was dismayed by her work history and reported that her substance use significantly interfered with her ability to find work, and she continued to believe that she had trouble finding work because of her former substance use, although she was vague about the connection.

Ms. Sanchez's physical and medical history includes falling and hitting her head on a rock when she was 4 years old. She reported frequent childhood nosebleeds and several head injuries from domestic violence, as well as a broken arm and a fractured nose. She reported being involved in violent relationships with her partners, as well as her pimp. She also stated that she had sustained a head injury in her 20s when she was pregnant and her partner hit her with a metal cane, knocking her unconscious and resulting in headaches for the following year. She described another instance of being beaten by the same boyfriend and pointed to a scar on her forehead, which she said was caused by his ring. Currently, she reports high blood pressure, fatigue, and headaches, in addition to pain throughout her body. Medical records indicate a long-standing history of dysthymia. She is currently taking medication for depression and fibromyalgia. Her medications include tramadol (25 mg qid [four times a day]), duloxetine (20 mg bid [twice a day]), and gabapentin (300 mg tid [three times a day]).

You have decided to give Ms. Sanchez a battery of tests to answer the referral question. During the testing, Ms. Sanchez was friendly, cooperative, and motivated. It took three sessions to complete the testing, and each session lasted approximately three hours. Ms. Sanchez rescheduled one session because of feeling ill. She appeared neatly groomed, wearing casual attire during the first testing session. During the second testing session, she wore a blouse with only the middle button buttoned, exposing a part of her breasts. During the third session, she wore short shorts and a tank top.

During the session, Ms. Sanchez appeared oriented to person, place, and time and thought content was appropriate to affect. During the first testing session, her comments were responsive, although you noticed it was challenging to develop an effective professional relationship with her because she was slightly withdrawn and, especially initially, she provided monosyllabic responses to questions. During the second and third sessions, she was increasingly verbally responsive to your comments, questions, and directions, although she also became more flirtatious in her interactions with you.

Ms. Sanchez did state that during the administration of the Wechsler Adult Intelligence Scale—Fourth Edition (WAIS–IV; Wechsler, 2008), she heard a voice telling her not to listen to your instructions and commented on your attractiveness. She stated that although she tried to block out the voice, it was difficult for her to concentrate. You provided frequent breaks during the testing in an attempt to maintain an acceptable level of attention, concentration, and performance.

Ms. Sanchez's affect was labile during the three testing sessions, ranging from depressed and tearful to euthymic. At the beginning of the first testing session and during some subtests of the WAIS—IV when she experienced difficulty, Ms. Sanchez was very tearful. In addition, she was tearful recounting her personal history in the second session. During all sessions, she complained of pain in her arms, hands, and legs and appeared to experience pain and walk with difficulty during breaks in testing.

Psychological Testing

You wanted to measure both personality and cognitive functioning. Therefore, you administered the following tests:

- Beck Depression Inventory—II (BDI–II; Beck, Steer, & Brown, 1996),
- Minnesota Multiphasic Personality Inventory—2 (MMPI–2; Butcher, Dahlstrom, Graham, Tellegen, & Kaemmer, 1989),
- Repeatable Battery for the Assessment of Neuropsychological Status (RBANS Update; Randolph, 2012),
- Trailmaking Test A and B (Army Individual Test Battery, 1944; Reitan & Wolfson, 1993),

- WAIS–IV, and
- Logical Memory I & II and Designs I & II from the Wechsler Memory Scales—Fourth Edition (WMS–IV; Wechsler, 2009).

Test Results

GENERAL INTELLECTUAL FUNCTIONING

Ms. Sanchez's WAIS–IV Full Scale IQ measured at 75 (5th percentile), which is within the borderline range of intellectual functioning. She obtained a scaled score of 80 on the Verbal Comprehension subscales, which measure general verbal abilities and abstract verbal reasoning (9th percentile), although her perceptual reasoning score was 70 (2nd percentile). Her performance was found to be lower than the IQ in the psychological record approximately four years ago, which was estimated to be in the Low Average Range, based on the Shipley Institute of Living Scale (Shipley-2). Although her overall IQ was low, her areas of relative strength were in verbal comprehension and expression. Ms. Sanchez had more difficulty with visuospatial tasks, including both visual comprehension and reasoning.

COGNITIVE FUNCTIONING

On the RBANS, which is a brief screen of cognitive functioning, Ms. Sanchez displayed performance in the borderline range, consistent with her intellectual abilities, in attention and concentration, immediate and delayed verbal memory abilities, and picture naming. She showed somewhat more impairment (at or below the 2nd percentile) in constructional abilities, including fine motor skills, visual perception, and visual memory.

On the Logical Memory I & II of the WMS–IV, Ms. Sanchez scored in the low average range of performance, slightly higher than expected, given her general intellectual level. On the Designs subtest, her performance was within the impaired range (1st percentile) in both immediate and delayed memory, with some improvement in recognition memory (5th percentile), although not statistically significantly higher than immediate and delayed memory and still within the borderline range of performance.

On measures of executive functioning, she consistently had difficulties. On both the Matrix Reasoning and Visual Puzzles subtests of the WAIS–IV, she scored below the 1st percentile. On the Trailmaking Test B, a measure of mental flexibility and the ability to understand the essential nature of a problem-solving task, she also scored below the 1st percentile.

PERSONALITY/EMOTIONAL FACTORS

The validity indicators on the MMPI-2 reflected a significant degree of emotional distress, although still within the range considered psychometrically valid. A scale that can reflect the degree of psychological resources available to deal with problems was very low. The scale measuring unusual experiences was high, although in a range that can be reflective more of general distress than an exaggeration of the problems present. Other validity scales that reflect an attempt to exaggerate or simulate, or indicate a specific tendency to respond in the positive to questions about psychopathology or to respond randomly, were not elevated. As a result, the validity of the testing results was adequate.

The highest clinical scale reflected strong feelings of depression, supported by her score of 33 on the BDI-II. The MMPI-2 codetype reflected a depressed person who is ruminatively introspective and evidences excessive indecision, doubts, and worry. She is likely to be obsessional about her own inadequacies and feels overwhelmed and extremely vulnerable. She may get so caught up in her internal thoughts, which can be not only intrusive but also disorganized, that she gets behaviorally paralyzed. It is not surprising that she has difficulty concentrating, in part perhaps because she easily becomes distracted by her own thinking. She likely experiences little pleasure from a life that is very challenging to her. Suicidality is always a major concern for a person with this type of profile. Ms. Sanchez probably has a tendency to overreact to minor stressors with agitation, guilt, and feelings of insecurity and inadequacy. She seems to have difficulty advocating for herself, instead responding to others with passivity and feelings of inferiority, increasing the likelihood that she will be taken advantage of. Her history of being exploited by others is reflected in mild elevation on the scale that measures paranoid thinking, reflecting her suspicion and mistrust of others. She admits to being socially isolated, and she presents as lacking in effective social skills. Perhaps because of her history of exploitative and ineffective interpersonal relationships, she is likely a person who feels lonely even when she is around others. The scale that can reflect psychotic thinking showed some degree of elevation. Given the multidimensional nature of that scale, the noted elevation could be an indication of the auditory hallucinations Ms. Sanchez periodically experiences, as well as a general sense of social alienation; alienation from herself; and her fears of losing control, both interpersonally and over her own internal life. A scale that measures concerns about physical health also showed mild elevation, which may reflect an attempt to manage her anxieties through focusing on physical dysfunction, although those attempts do not appear to be successful.

Assessment Considerations

This case is quite different from the other two cases, especially John Smith (see Chapter 5, this volume), because we already have a considerable amount of information, even though not as much as would be ideal. We know the purpose and goal of this assessment because they were stated clearly in the referral from the attorney. So the goal, in this case, would be to write a formal report for the referring attorney with specific answers to the question posed.

The first question that should occur to you is, What are the sources of information you should look for to answer the referral question? If you need to, look back at our discussion of sources of information in Chapter 3. Certainly, you would want to do a fairly extensive clinical interview. That is the core of any assessment process, whether formal, which usually ends with a written report, or informal, as part of a psychotherapeutic assessment process. Observing the person's behaviors and, perhaps, asking specific questions regarding mentation are integral parts of any interview, so those two sources of data will certainly be included. The referral was made to you as a psychologist, so use of psychological tests, one of the unique areas of practice for psychologists, will also be important, in our opinion. As is typical in a referral from an attorney, multiple records are available: medical, prison, legal, and psychological. At this point we might defer a decision about collateral interviews. The two most important questions here are, Whom might you interview? and, What specific information would you hope to get from collateral sources? Those questions should also be answered before proceeding with any collateral interviews.

Given that the case, as provided, includes a considerable amount of test data, a number of questions arise about the tests used. Normally, you would want to have answers to the questions we discuss below before you even consider which tests to administer.

What types of tests are relevant in this case? The term *mental impairment* is pretty nonspecific. If that is as specific as the referral question is, you need to think of a number of possibilities. First, Ms. Sanchez could have limited intellectual ability, which makes it difficult for her to function independently. To find that out, a test of intellectual functioning would be appropriate. Or she could be experiencing some kind of acquired brain dysfunction, such as a disease that affects brain tissue; common examples would be a brain tumor or a cerebral vascular accident (stroke) or a brain injury, such as a head trauma. We do have evidence from her medical record of a number of head injuries. What we do not know with much specificity is how severe any damage to her brain might have been, whether there were any behavioral or cognitive sequelae (results or consequences), and how long term any such effects may have been.

Sometimes, although not always, a closer review of medical records can provide some answers, but rarely do medical records provide much in the way of psychological (cognitive, emotional, behavioral) information regarding head injuries. Beyond the records, tests that evaluate brain functioning, that is, neuropsychological tests, would provide helpful information.

The case description suggests that Ms. Sanchez reports reported feelings of sadness and lack of energy, with some suicidal ideation, stress, difficulty concentrating, and poor memory. The latter two cognitive symptoms, which might affect her abilities to function independently, could be the result of some kind of brain dysfunction, or they could also be the result of stress and depression. So, some kind of measure of her psychological functioning, that is, personality testing, is indicated. We do not know the exact nature of her psychological issues, so a test that measures a broad range of psychological dysfunction would be most useful. Ms. Sanchez goes on to report auditory hallucinations, so a personality test that measures psychotic symptoms would be important. She also complains of vague symptoms of fatigue and pain. A number of medical illnesses can cause such symptoms, but it is also the case that people who want to present in an overly negative manner, in this case possibly as a means of gaining a financial advantage by qualifying for a federal supplemental income program, can also present with vague symptoms of fatigue and pain. So, measures that evaluate the tendency to exaggerate or simulate psychological or physical symptoms would be essential, as well as making sure that she has had a recent assessment by a physician to determine the current medical contributions to such symptoms. She also reports a history of polysubstance abuse, so some measure of chemical dependency is necessary, even though she reports being sober for more than 2 years. The fact that she is experiencing stress in her life increases the risk that she might return to the use of chemicals as a means of self-medication. It is important that as a professional psychologist you neither make assumptions about people before you have collected the requisite data nor accept what others report to you at face value. It is not that you should not trust others but that you need to verify everything you possibly can. If you do not, at some point in your career you will be caught assuming something that is not true. At best, it will be embarrassing to you; at worst, it will be harmful to those you work with.

So, at this point you are thinking that you want measures of intellectual function, personality dysfunction, neuropsychological functioning, and chemical dependency. You know one thing from observations during the interview, which is rich with possible causes: Ms. Sanchez had difficulty reporting facts accurately. You will want to consider (i.e., collect data about) a number of etiologies for such a presentation, including psychotic thinking, memory difficulties, lack of verbal skill, or lack of engagement in the assessment process. That is a fairly inclusive list of problems to evaluate and should provide the basis to answer the referral question. The next question you should ask yourself is whether you are the appropriate person to undertake this assessment, and if yes, whether you are going to take it all on. You are fairly new in your private practice (in the described scenario), so you may well feel a temptation to take on all comers. That is a very bad idea. That is especially true when the referral comes from an attorney. Not many experiences that psychologists have are more sobering than being grilled on the witness stand by the opposing attorney and being shown to be lacking in competence or knowledge about something you have done. As a colleague has quipped,

> Be gratified by the knowledge of what you know. Strive to know
> that which you know you don't know. Don't worry about the
> many things you don't know you don't know. These things
> will be called to your attention by a cross-examining attorney.
> (D. Martindale, personal communication, July 31, 2014)

Most psychologists have had considerable training in assessing intellectual functioning and personality dysfunction, so you probably have had such training (remember, for the purposes of this example, you are now a licensed psychologist). The question here is whether now, 3 years after your obtained your degree, you have continued to be active enough in those areas, both in terms of continuing to practice in those areas and of staying current with the literature in those areas, to be competent to provide assessment in those two areas. Fewer psychologists have had training in neuropsychology. If you have had no such training, don't do it!

If you are clear with your referral sources about the boundaries of your competence, they will learn whom to refer to you and whom to refer elsewhere. And if they are the kind of referral sources you want, they will respect you for your honesty about your competencies. That does not mean that a screening for brain functioning is inappropriate— again, assuming you have some training and experience in doing so. A screening can provide sufficient data regarding whether a referral should be made for a more complete neuropsychological assessment. Perhaps even fewer psychologists have had much training, with supervision, in assessing chemical dependency. If you decide you are not competent in that area, you should refer.

Once you have decided which problem areas you have the competency to assess and you have decided which general types of tests would be appropriate in this case, you need to ask yourself which specific tests you want to use. The following should be viewed as simply illustrative of the thinking process you should go through. You made choices on certain tests (some of which we discuss below), but other tests could have been used and might even have been more appropriate.

As we stated in Chapter 3, this volume, the first and most important questions you should ask yourself regarding the use of any specific test is whether the test being considered is valid for the purpose and the person being tested, that is, Has research been conducted to ensure that this test has adequate reliability and validity for the population of people from whom the specific examinee comes? The manual for the test should provide helpful information on the norms developed and the standardization sample used. The latter information will tell you whether the test fits the person you have in mind to test. Because the manual was created by the publisher, it would be wise to consult a more independent evaluation of the test. Two excellent sources are *Buros Mental Measurement Yearbook* (Carlson, Geisinger, & Jonson, 2014) and *Tests in Print*, also published by Buros (Murphy, Geisinger, Carlson, & Spies, 2011).

To measure intellectual functioning, you used the WAIS–IV in this assessment. The Wechsler tests are among the most widely used tests of intelligence. The WAIS–IV has well-documented data on reliability and validity for use with individuals with Ms. Sanchez's age, language, socioeconomic, gender, and ethnic background (Wechsler, 2008). One disadvantage is that it is not based on a widely accepted theory of intellectual functioning, such as the Cattell–Horn–Carroll theory (Flanagan & Harrison, 2005; McGrew & Flanagan, 1998). That theory serves as the basis for the most recent editions of the Woodcock–Johnson test (Schrank, Mather, & McGrew, 2014) and Stanford–Binet Intelligence Scales (Roid, 2003), which would also be good choices to use with a person like Ms. Sanchez. Among other tests that could provide a valid assessment of her intellectual abilities are the Kaufman Adolescent and Adult Intelligence Test (Kaufman & Kaufman, 1993), the Cognitive Assessment System 2nd Ed. (Naglieri, Das, & Goldstein, 2014), and the Differential Abilities Scale (Elliott, 2007).

You also chose a general measure of psychological dysfunction. You know from the case history that these include symptoms of depression, possible psychotic thinking, and paranoid thinking. With regard to the latter symptom, remember that paranoia can be based on reality—to wit, the saying from Joseph Heller's (1961) delightful, satirical novel, *Catch-22*: "Just because you're paranoid doesn't mean they aren't after you."

You chose the MMPI–2 because it is the most widely used and researched test of psychopathology. Literally thousands of studies have been done, initially on the MMPI (Hathaway & McKinley, 1942) and subsequently on the MMPI–2, which was first published in 1989 (Graham, 1990). Using this test with Ms. Sanchez has an excellent empirical basis. An advantage of the MMPI–2 is that it provides measures of all of the suspected areas of psychological dysfunction, including depression, psychosis, and paranoia, plus it provides an assessment of interpersonal skill and involvement, which could be a contributing problem for Ms. Sanchez, and it provides measures of test-taking approach, that is, it gives you some basis for knowing whether she is exaggerating or underreporting the extent of her psychological problems. Alternative measures of general psychopathology could be used. A particularly good choice would be the Personality Assessment Inventory developed by Morey (1991), also an increasingly widely used test that was developed using more modern test construction methods and that has categories that are more closely aligned with the *International Statistical Classification of Diseases and Related Health Problems* (ICD–10; World Health Organization [WHO], 2016) than are the MMPI–2 scales. You also administered the BDI–II. The assessment basis for using this test is only moderately strong, as it is not as reliable a test as the depression scales on the MMPI–2, but it takes little time for either examinee or psychologist, so the cost is not high. If it provides similar results to the MMPI–2, it provides a bit more confidence in the results. If the score is different, however, it creates a problem of what to do with the results. Most often, one would trust the MMPI–2 more than the BDI–II, meaning that it adds only mild incremental value.

You decided to do a neuropsychological screening but not a complete neuropsychological assessment. One relatively brief general measure of neuropsychological functioning was used, the RBANS Update, and the Trailmaking Test, as the RBANS Update does not have a good measure of executive functioning. The WAIS–IV does provide some measure of executive functioning, but having an additional, independent measure of it for convergence is a good idea. In addition, the WMS–IV subscales of Logical Memory and Designs are useful measures of memory for stories and for spatial figures. The Logical Memory scales measure the kinds of information people normally come across in daily life, information about situations, as opposed to a shopping list, for example; the Designs scales measure memory for an unfamiliar spatial design, a somewhat more pure visual task compared with the visual memory component of the RBANS Update, so you get two slightly different measures of this ability. You decided on the addition of a test of memory because of specific questions during the interview about her memory abilities. However, because you did not feel competent to do a complete neuropsychological assessment, you also entertained the possibility of a referral for a complete neuropsychological assessment, depending on the data obtained from the tests that you administered.

You also did not feel comfortable doing a chemical dependency assessment. Thus, you recommended to the attorney that a referral for a chemical dependency assessment be made.

Let us take a brief look at the data again to see what conclusions we can draw, with regard both to the ultimate referral question and what additional testing might be necessary, if any.

First, from the interview, you know Ms. Sanchez is of Mexican American heritage, so the effects ethnicity can have on the reliability and validity of psychological tools, as well as her personal and interpersonal functioning, will need to be kept in mind.

She has had a very challenging life, with the early death of her father and a nonsupportive mother who was overwhelmed with the responsibilities of her family after her husband died. To assist the family financially, Ms. Sanchez dropped out of school and turned to prostitution, with few other avenues available to her, and began using drugs and alcohol. She has two children, of whom she does not have custody.

When she was in her early 20s, she received her GED and attempted to further her education, unsuccessfully. She has worked in multiple jobs, suggesting limited effectiveness or lack of ability to stick to one position. On the positive side, she reports having been drug free for more than 2 years, although that has not yet been conclusively established. Some clarification of current drug use and its potential impact on her employability should be part of the referral question to a chemical dependency specialist.

Ms. Sanchez reports feeling unhappy, with lack of energy and difficulty concentrating. She sleeps most afternoons and describes some suicidal ideation but without current intent or plan.

She reports a series of head traumas, whose consequences are unclear. She complains of vague medical symptoms, which could be the result of fibromyalgia, or depression, or could be the result of the conversion of psychological distress into medical complaints. All possibilities should be considered. However, it should be noted that the question about which might best explain her physical symptoms is not a referral question. When responding to a referral from an attorney, in particular, it is far better just to respond to the questions asked, rather than questions that are not asked. Keeping in mind that her medical problems could have a relationship with psychological issues, however, might help you understand Ms. Sanchez better. (For a summary of the psychological issues in fibromyalgia, see White, Nielson, Harth, Ostbye, & Speechley, 2002.)

You noticed a general willingness to be cooperative and motivation to respond appropriately and with sufficient care to the psychological tests. She was adequately oriented times three (appropriately aware of person, place, and time), but she also reported hearing a voice telling her not to listen to your instructions. She demonstrated a range of emotional reactions, with some emotional lability. During the second and third sessions, Ms. Sanchez acted in a sexually provocative and flirtatious manner.

The WAIS–IV results indicate that Ms. Sanchez is a person with limited intellectual ability. An important question is whether the scores on the WAIS–IV and the previous Shipley-2 are statistically significantly different (i.e., no overlap in the confidence intervals of each score based on the respective standard error of the measurements) or whether this is a case of variability in scores that is within the expected range. Whichever is the case, generally one would place more confidence in the WAIS–IV score because the reliability measures on this test are superior to those on the Shipley-2.

The results on the RBANS Update indicated that Ms. Sanchez performed with mild impairment only in visual perception, visual memory retrieval, and constructional abilities. With cues, her visual memory did improve. Her performance on tests of executive functioning—the ability to plan, organize, and strategize—were consistently in the impaired range.

From the MMPI–2, we have indications that the psychological test data are adequately valid, although they reflect a high degree of general psychological distress. Knowing that is an important place to start before attempting to draw any conclusions from the specific testing data. From the MMPI–2 and the BDI–II, we have data that suggest a moderate to severe level of depression, with difficulties in interpersonal relationships, and a high level of unusual experiences that can point to psychotic thinking, although her depression seems to be primary and may drive her auditory hallucinations. A person with this level of emotional distress and agitation will almost always have difficulties with concentration and attention. Hence, it is very difficult to know whether her cognitive difficulties are a result of psychological or neurological factors. What is almost certainly the case is that her limited intellectual abilities and possible brain dysfunction, perhaps as a result of repeated head injuries or chemical use, make it more difficult for her to cope with and manage a life that would be challenging for most of us.

Now, let us return to the question of collateral interviews. On two bases, pursuing that source of data does not seem necessary. First, the data you have obtained seem to provide a fairly consistent picture of Ms. Sanchez, leaving questions you cannot answer regarding brain functioning and chemical dependency because you do not have the expertise, but otherwise the results seem pretty clear. Second, there does not appear to be anyone you could consult to get a clearer picture of her.

Diagnostic Considerations

The diagnostic process is much easier with ample data from a variety of sources, especially when those sources of data agree with each other. Thus, unlike the cases in Chapters 4 and 5, this case offers a better opportunity for you to come to a definitive diagnosis. You have convergent data from Ms. Sanchez's self-description, behavioral observations, medical records, and psychological test data that she is experiencing a moderate to severe level of depression. Thus, a diagnosis of depression seems fairly self-evident. The major question would be, What form of depression does she have? Given the medical record statement about a long history of dysthymia, it does not seem to be a Major depressive episode, single episode (F32). The medical record points to a Dysthymic disorder (F34.1), but the psychological test data and observations, supported by her self-report, suggest a more severe level of depression. You have seen no evidence of cycling into mania (i.e., Bipolar disorder; F31). Hence, the best diagnosis for Ms. Sanchez appears to be Major depressive disorder, recurrent (F33). The remaining question in that regard is what to do with her auditory hallucinations. One possibility is to give her a dual diagnosis of major depression and psychosis, with the latter being (a) a Delusional disorder (F22), although the *Blue Book* (WHO, 1993) states that clear and persistent auditory hallucinations are incompatible with this diagnosis (p. 85); (b) a Brief psychotic disorder (F23), which, however, requires an acute onset within the previous 2 weeks (*Blue Book*, p. 8); or perhaps most suitably, (c) a Schizoaffective disorder, depressive type (F25.1), although the voices do not appear to engage in a running commentary on Ms. Sanchez's behavior or to have a discussion among various voices about her (as suggested by the *Blue Book* [pp. 78, 91] guideline on hallucinations).

However, two factors mitigate against that type of dual diagnosis, that is, some kind of depressive disorder plus some kind of psychotic disorder. First, the Clinical Modification of the ICD–10 (ICD–10–CM; National Center for Health Statistics, 2015) does not allow for such dual diagnoses. No diagnosis of a severe major depression is independent of psychotic features. That is, with a severe major depression, one has to choose either with psychotic symptoms (F33.3) or without psychotic symptoms (F33.2). It would not be logical to choose F33.2, then add F22 or F25.1 as an additional diagnosis, and the code F33.3 already includes both her depression and hallucinations. Second, it does appear that Ms. Sanchez's depression is the primary diagnostic feature, with the auditory hallucinations all revolving around it, with the voice's messages centering around self-harm or social interaction. Therefore, a primary diagnosis of Major depressive disorder, recurrent, severe with psychotic symptoms (F33.3) is the most appropriate one. Most of her reported symptoms fall well within this diagnosis, constant sadness, difficulty concentrating, low energy level, poor memory, and fatigue.

Some of those symptoms also fit other diagnostic categories that should be considered. We know from the medical record that she has been diagnosed with Fibromyalgia (M79.7). Many of her symptoms of fibromyalgia (fatigue and pain, in particular) could also be the result of her depression. However, not only is it not necessary for you to try to change her diagnosis from fibromyalgia to depression but also, as a non-physician, it would be inappropriate for you to do so. There is one other interesting consideration related to her diagnosis of fibromyalgia. Often, you can note the medications a person is taking as an indication of the diagnosis given that person by a physician. In this case, Ms. Sanchez is taking duloxetine (Cymbalta), a serotonin–norepinephrine reuptake inhibitor commonly used for the treatment of depression. Aha! The physician's treatment provides support for your diagnosis of depression! However, alas, duloxetine is also used to treat pain (remember, pain is also mediated by the serotonin neurotransmitter system), so is a common pharmacological treatment for fibromyalgia. So, beware of using the record of medications to point you to a specific diagnosis.

Some of the symptoms can also be the result of an abnormality in brain functioning, especially concentration, memory, and headaches. You have some testing data to support difficulties with concentration and attention, visual memory recall, and executive functioning. However, you are not a trained neuropsychologist, so you have recommended referral for a more complete neuropsychological assessment. Nevertheless, you can get a *rule-out diagnosis*, which is a hypothesized diagnosis for which additional data are necessary. You have the best evidence for a memory disorder. To consider this as a primary diagnosis, you have to move out of Chapter 5 of the ICD–10–CM ("Mental, Behavioral, and Neurodevelopmental Disorders"), which includes the diagnoses we have discussed up to the point. Memory disorders are found in the other section of the ICD–10–CM that is most often used by psychologists, Chapter 18 ("Symptoms, Signs, and Abnormal Clinical and Laboratory Findings"), not elsewhere classified, and more specifically to the section Symptoms and Signs Involving Cognition, Perception, Emotional State and Behavior. Here the *Blue Book* is not going to be of any assistance, as it discusses only the diagnoses in Chapter 5. Consultation with another text on psychopathology would be recommended.

So, which diagnoses should you consider from Chapter 18 in the ICD–10–CM? You know that Ms. Sanchez has difficulty retrieving new memories, although she was able to describe her past life adequately, so Anterograde amnesia (R41.1) makes the most sense, although Other amnesia (R41.3), which includes Amnesia NOS and Memory loss NOS, are also possible diagnoses. We know that her cognitive problems go beyond memory impairment, however, so one might also provide rule-out diagnoses of Mild cognitive impairment, so stated (G31.84); Intracranial injury (S06); or Other specified mental disorders due to known physiological condition (F06.8), which can include mild memory impairment, although the only evidence you have for that diagnosis is the history of head injuries, the severity and impact of which you know very little. Last, Alcohol dependence with alcohol-induced persisting amnestic disorder (F10.26) or Alcohol use with alcohol-induced persisting amnestic disorder (F10.96) should certainly be a rule-out diagnosis until you have additional information from the chemical dependency evaluation.

Now, back to the original referral question: Is Ms. Sanchez impaired? Is she able to work? What do you think?

First and foremost, that is a very difficult question to answer as a psychologist, and psychologists should be careful to address only those areas in which we have competence. Most psychologists are not employment specialists, so we do not know all of the skills necessary to be gainfully employed. So, providing a definitive answer to the question is likely beyond the competence of most of us, unless we have had specialized training and experience in the field of employment assessment.

What you can say, however, is that Ms. Sanchez faces a variety of challenges that have made it difficult for her to maintain employment and are likely to play a role in her future employment. What are those challenges? First, she has limited intellectual abilities and limited educational preparation, so only nonskilled work would be an option for her. Second, she has some cognitive difficulties that would challenge her ability to do unskilled work. Her verbal skills are adequate, such that she might even appear more skilled than she is, but her visuospatial skills are generally very poor, including her fine motor skills. Thus, a task that requires her to use her visual perception and motor skills, such as assembly line work, would likely be very difficult for her. Third, beyond her cognitive limitations, her psychological status adds to her challenges. Her depression causes her to have a low energy level, low motivation, and difficulties with concentration, all of which would make it difficult for her to engage in exactly the kind of task her intellectual abilities make appropriate for her, namely, a repetitive, physical task. Finally, her family background and responsibilities have added an additional layer of stress to her life, which, combined with her limited resources, may have resulted in her feeling overwhelmed. Certainly, she did not have the social and emotional support that she needed to cope effectively.

Given all of these challenges and her difficulty with planning and organizing (executive functions), especially with spatial tasks, anything more than a repetitive, assembly-line type task will be beyond her cognitive and psychological abilities. Add to that the pain she experiences as a result of her fibromyalgia, and there are very few jobs she would be able to hold over time, which is exactly what her history demonstrates. Bottom line: Due to this complex set of factors, it would be difficult to be the employment specialist whose job it is to find an appropriate job for her. In this case, your task is to help the employment specialist by describing Ms. Sanchez's problems and explaining something of the difficulties that she experiences that affect her ability to carry out tasks. This is another reminder for you to restrict yourself to your area of expertise, that is, emotions, cognitions, and behaviors.

Closing Comments

The cases of Lynn, John Smith, and Anne Sanchez raise a number of questions about assessment and diagnosis and determining the procedures to conduct a thorough assessment and arrive at a diagnosis. These tasks can feel daunting, particularly if you are fairly new at the process of psychological assessment and diagnosis. Never fear! One of the authors of this text remembers a very early supervision session in graduate school during which the supervisor asked him, in response to something he had said to the patient during the second session with her, what his case conceptualization was at that point. He replied that he was struggling to understand what the person's experience was and could not do that and think about case conceptualization at the same time. The supervisor helpfully stated that with experience, the ability to listen and think conceptually at the same time would come. And, it did!

Ethics of Assessment— Protecting Your Patients

7

Although we have presented ethical discussions throughout this text, in this chapter we specifically explore ethical considerations in conducting assessments and arriving at diagnoses. It is not possible for a conscientious psychologist to divorce ethics from other aspects of practice. Ethics is foundational to the practice of psychology and permeates all our professional behavior. So, although we consider ethics separately in this chapter as a means of providing a more comprehensive and reasonably succinct overview of the ethical issues involved in psychological assessments, you (as a student of psychology) should think about these issues as being embedded in every aspect of what we as psychologists do.

The major ethical question that has confronted humans, perhaps from the time they attained consciousness, has been, What is the right thing to do? In other words, What does it mean to be virtuous in this situation, with these people, with this set of circumstances (MacIntyre, 1998)? The quest for

http://dx.doi.org/10.1037/14778-008

A Student's Guide to Assessment and Diagnosis Using the ICD–10–CM: Psychological and Behavioral Conditions, by J. Schaffer and E. Rodolfa the correct answers to that question has been the focus of moral philosophy since at least the time of the Greek writer and philosopher Homer about 3,000 years ago. The answers to the questions are, however, culture bound, as is most of what people think and believe. For Homer, the right thing was for a person to perform "his socially allotted function" (MacIntyre, 1998, p. 8), which for most men at the time meant technical skill (especially military), courage, cunning, and aggressiveness, and for married women it meant being faithful in marriage (MacIntyre, 1998)—at the time, few other attributes were important for women! Clearly and thankfully, the view of what constitutes the right thing to do, or virtue, has changed considerably since that time. So, how does one decide today what the right thing to do as a psychologist is?

For most psychologists in North America, the standards by which we make that judgment professionally are grounded in the *Ethical Principles of Psychologists and Code of Conduct* (hereinafter, Ethics Code) of the American Psychological Association (APA, 2010) and the *Canadian Code of Ethics for Psychologists* (hereinafter, Code; Canadian Psychological Association, 2000). In addition to standards for professional conduct in specific situations, both codes also provide general guidelines for how one thinks about and approaches ethical behavior by enumerating certain guiding principles for ethical behavior (see Exhibit 7.1 and Exhibit 7.2). To some degree, these principles are aspirational in nature. They set goals toward which an ethical psychologist should strive. However, both codes also spell out specific, minimal ethical standards (i.e., the minimum level of ethical behavior that is acceptable for a psychologist) to which a psychologist is expected to adhere. We provide a brief summary of the principles here, and we reference specific standards throughout the remainder of this chapter, but every student of psychology and every practicing psychologist should at least be familiar with the code of their home country.

The principles enumerated in the ethics codes of the APA and the CPA are similar, although packaged somewhat differently. The APA Ethics

---

EXHIBIT 7.1

Ethical Principles From *Ethical Principles of Psychologists and Code of Conduct* (American Psychological Association, 2010)

Principle A: Beneficence and Nonmaleficence
Principle B: Fidelity and Responsibility
Principle C: Integrity
Principle D: Justice
Principle E: Respect for People's Rights and Dignity

EXHIBIT 7.2

**Ethical Principles From *Canadian Code of Ethics for Psychologists*
(Canadian Psychological Association, 2000)**

Principle I: Respect for the Dignity of Persons
Principle II: Responsible Caring
Principle III: Integrity in Relationships
Principle IV: Responsibility to Society

Code lists the following principles that serve as the foundation of ethical behavior:

- *Principle A: Beneficence and Nonmaleficence*, that is, striving to benefit those with whom we work and taking care to do no harm, recognizing that our own needs and biases can interfere with providing help and avoiding harm, and actively looking for ways in which harm can occur. As ethical psychologists, we proactively take steps to minimize harmful outcomes and maximize benefits, including ensuring competence in our activities and self-reflective consideration of our actions and motives.

- *Principle B: Fidelity and Responsibility* involves behaviors necessary to establish professional relationships of trust, including being aware of professional responsibilities to society and professional communities, upholding professional standards, accepting responsibility for our behavior, and seeking to manage conflicts that can lead to harm or exploitation. It is our ethical responsibility to work collaboratively with other professionals when it in the best interest of our clients.

- *Principle C: Integrity* emphasizes promoting truthfulness and honesty in practice of psychology, and striving to follow through on commitments and obligations.

- *Principle D: Justice* recognizes the rights of others and provides us with a guideline regarding exercising sound judgment in the practice of psychology. We recognize potential biases, manage boundaries of practice, and acknowledge that all individuals are entitled to access to the contributions that the field of psychology provides.

- *Principle E: Respect for People's Rights and Dignity* involves respecting the dignity and worth of all people and the rights individuals have to privacy, confidentiality, and self-determination, respecting the breadth of cultural and individual differences and neither participating in nor condoning activities based on prejudice.

One helpful feature that the CPA Code provides is a rank ordering of the weight that should be given to the various principles when a particular situation results in a conflict between the principles, that is, when one cannot follow one principle without being in violation of another. An example of such a conflict is provided below, following the ordering of principles by the CPA Code. They are as follows:

- *Principle I: Respect for the Dignity of Persons* is the rights of the individual to be treated with respect as a person with worth and to certain considerations, including privacy, self-determination, personal liberty, and justice, with special responsibility to those most vulnerable.
- *Principle II: Responsible Caring* is an active caring for the welfare of others, including the concepts of beneficence and nonmaleficence, emphasizing that we, as psychologists, should strive to benefit those with whom we work and taking care to do no harm, recognizing that our own needs and biases can interfere with providing help and avoiding harm, and actively looking for ways in which harm can occur and proactively taking steps to minimize harmful outcomes and maximize benefits, including ensuring competence in our activities and self-reflective consideration of our actions and motives.
- *Principle III: Integrity in Relationships* involves (a) establishing relationships of trust and (b) acting in ways that promote honesty, accuracy, straightforwardness, openness, and truthfulness, including maintaining standards of conduct, making clear what the professional role involves, accepting responsibility for our own behaviors, minimizing bias, and avoiding conflicts of interest.
- *Principle IV: Responsibility to Society* is a commitment to fairness and justice, not only in professional relationships but in society, including equal access to services offered by psychologists and knowledge created by psychological research.

We emphasize that the order of these principles does not suggest that the later principles are less important to the practice of psychology, only that the first principles take precedent when the principles conflict.

The principles from the two ethics codes reflect the history of Western moral philosophy in a number of ways (MacIntyre, 1998). First, the codes reflect the tension between individualism and communalism. On the one hand, each psychologist is responsible for choosing between various ethical options, and further, individuals (including psychologists) have the freedom and the power to make choices. Our behaviors are not totally determined, and we must take responsibility for the choices we make. At the same time there is a concern for the broader social community, a perspective that was core to early Greek thinking regarding morality and responsibility. Both codes reflect the responsibility that we have toward the larger human community, in particular, our responsibility to advocate for justice and fairness, in addition to our primary responsibility for our clients, whether individuals, groups, or organizations, with whom we work. We also emphasize that the codes address our behaviors and roles as psychologists, not our broader moral responsibilities to each other as individuals.

Second, the principles of the codes reflect a concern for the other and the human rights of all persons: "Psychologists respect the dignity and worth of all people, and the rights of individuals to privacy, confidentiality, and self-determination" (APA Ethics Code, p. 4) and each person has dignity and the right to "privacy, self-determination, personal liberty, and natural justice" (CPA Code, p. 8). These rights can only be abridged by a contractual agreement between the individual and the other party, whether that party is the state or an individual, such as a psychologist. The primary goal of ethical behavior is the well-being of those with whom we work, and in particular those most vulnerable, as opposed to choosing behaviors based on how we can benefit from the relationship (see, by comparison, Machiavelli, 1532/2008).

The process of diagnosis has important ethical implications. To the degree that an incorrect diagnosis from the Clinical Modification of the *International Statistical Classification of Diseases and Related Health Problems* (ICD–10–CM; National Center for Health Statistics, 2015) is used, based on an inadequate or inappropriate assessment process, there may result an inaccurate understanding of the individual and resulting ill-advised or ineffective recommendations regarding disposition. With these introductory comments forming the foundation of our understanding of the ethical principles, we now turn our attention to the cases we have been discussing.

Case 1—Lynn

A number of primary ethical issues are associated with Case 1: testing, training, confidentiality, and mental health provider roles. Competence is also a concern, but we discuss this in Chapter 8.

Lynn was referred by her sister to a training clinic that had doctoral students as the primary service providers. To meet the requirements of an assessment course you were taking, you proposed to administer three psychological tests to Lynn. Is there a problem here? Students have a right to be trained adequately, do they not? And tests provide useful information, do they not? We said so ourselves in Chapter 3!

The problem lies primarily in the use of the three tests. First of a number of potential problems, are those tests necessary for the purposes of this psychological service? Let us deal with each test separately. Is there evidence of a psychological dysfunction for which the Minnesota Multiphasic Personality Inventory—2 (MMPI–2; Butcher, Dahlstrom, Graham, Tellegen, & Kaemmer, 1989), would be an appropriate assessment tool? Probably, yes. Lynn presents with depression and/or anxiety, for which the MMPI–2 could well provide useful information and for the identification of which the MMPI–2 was originally developed (Graham, 2000). In addition, Lynn falls into the category of individuals on which the MMPI–2 has been well normed, so the test would be used appropriately for the purposes for which it was designed. However, that leaves a number of questions that should be asked. First, is there a reasonable expectation that the MMPI–2 would provide useful information beyond that obtained through the clinical interview? Possibly, yes. Is there another test that might provide even better or more relevant information, without the length of the MMPI–2? Potentially, the answer is yes, for instance, the Personality Assessment Inventory (PAI; Morey, 1991), the NEO Personality Inventory—III (Costa & McCrae, 2005) or the California Personality Inventory—Revised (CPI–R; Gough, 1987), or the 16 Personality Factor Questionnaire (Cattell, Cattell, & Cattell, 2002)—and this view is held by both of the authors who are strong advocates of the MMPI–2. Who is going to pay for the administration, scoring, and interpretation of the test? If Lynn pays directly, is that a wise use of her funds? If a third-party payer (like an insurance company), are there limits to the amount the insurance company will pay, and if so, is it wise to use part of the reimbursement Lynn would get for psychological services for the MMPI–2? Does it add enough to make its use justified? None of this should be interpreted as an argument not to use the MMPI–2, but these are questions, of both a practical and ethical nature, that should be considered.

The use of the Millon Clinical Multiaxial Inventory—III (MCMI–III) is potentially more problematic. Why is this particular test being used on this particular person? That is a different question from why this test is being used as a required test in an assessment course. Ample evidence in the literature (Jankowski, 2002; Millon & Bloom, 2008; Strack, 2008) indicates that the MCMI–III was developed for the assessment of individuals with personality disorders. Is there any evidence in what we know now that Lynn has a personality disorder? Likely the answer is no. Then why is the MCMI–III being used? In addition to the general ethical guideline to use tests only for the purposes for which they were designed (APA Ethics Code, Standard 9.08(b); CPA Code, Ethical Standard II.21), a problem with the MCMI–III is that it should not be used as a screening tool for psychopathology (Craig, 1999; Millon & Bloom, 2008; R. Rogers, 2003). Virtually everyone, whether they have a personality disorder or not, is likely to have elevation on at least one scale of the MCMI–III (Millon & Bloom, 2008). The MCMI–III profile alone does not tell us whether that is a problem or, merely, a personality style. This is more true of the personality disorder scales than of the Axis I scales, although in Lynn's case, using the MCMI–III to distinguish between depression and anxiety has problems of its own (see Saulsman, 2011) and may not add anything to the information provided by the MMPI–2. As a result, it will be helpful to provide a clear rationale for the use of the MCMI–III that describes Lynn's specific needs and goals.

There is, perhaps, an even greater difficulty with the use of the Stanford–Binet Intelligence Scales (fifth ed.; SB5; Roid, 2003). What evidence do we have that intelligence may be an issue related to Lynn's presenting problems? What kind of information might the SB5 provide that can be expected to be of significant usefulness?

Given these questions/problems, what are the ethical concerns associated with your assessment plan? The first question, as described above, is whether the tests being used are appropriate for a person like Lynn (or, to use the more technical language, whether the test is reliable and valid for the purposes being used and whether it will provide useful information). The second question has to do with the purpose and goal of using these tests: Is the primary purpose for the benefit of Lynn or for your benefit, given that you need to complete a battery of tests using these three tests to meet course requirements? If the latter (which appears to be the case), how does that speak to the ethical requirement not to exploit a patient for the psychologist's own benefit (APA Ethics Code, Standard 3.08; CPA Code, Ethical Standard III.31)? Your being in a multiple relationship with Lynn (APA Ethics Code, Standard 3.05; CPA Code, Ethical Standards I.26, III.33, III.34) also carries the risk of your playing a role of being an evaluator/therapist and, at the same time, a graduate student who is asking Lynn for a favor, and/or a conflict of interest (APA Ethics Code, Standard 3.06; CPA Code, Ethical Standard III.31) whereby you are proposing a service that Lynn may not really need without adequate consideration of the impact that may have on her or the consequences of requesting Lynn to take these tests.

So, is the provision of services by students, who by definition have a lower level of competence than independently practicing psychologists, always unethical? In a word, no. And perhaps we should be more emphatic: Absolutely not!

Two factors can make provision of services by students ethical. First, services are offered only under supervision, so the student is receiving continual input regarding how best to provide the service and is not practicing independently (which would be not only an ethical violation but also a violation of the law regardless of the jurisdiction where the training takes place).

The second factor has to do with the nature of the interaction between student and client. The appropriate means for dealing with this dilemma in this context is based on the principles of respect, beneficence, and integrity and is focused on the process of informed consent (APA Ethics Code, Standards 3.10, 9.03, 10.01; CPA Code, Ethical Standards I.16–I.36). One can see even from the number of references to informed consent in the two ethics codes how important it is for psychologists. The ethical imperative is to provide full, open, and noncoercive informed consent and in turn assessment and/or treatment that allows the individual to make a voluntary and knowledgeable decision (Bersoff, DeMatteo, & Foster, 2012). This means having an open and honest discussion with a client about the goals of and reasons for all psychological services being proposed, along with a consideration of alternatives to the proposed services. In this case, if you seek to use the tests proposed to meet a class requirement (as well as to gain some potentially useful information), that purpose needs to be explained to Lynn and a discussion undertaken to make sure than Lynn understands and consents willingly. In other words, "getting" Lynn to sign a consent form is not adequate. But, beyond that, the goal should also not be simply obtaining her acquiescence. Patients are usually cooperative and go out of their way to be responsive to mental health professionals. Lynn needs to know that the choice is completely hers and that if she decides to decline, there will be no negative consequences, either in your feelings toward her or in the possible therapy offered in the future. And this process takes a good deal of self-knowledge and self-monitoring on your part. If you feel a strong need to meet your class requirement (and we, the authors, as current or former faculty, hope you do) and you have seen Lynn's situation as a perfect opportunity to do so, it will be a difficult task for you to prevent your disappointment in Lynn's declining to take the tests from getting in the way of your attitudes and behaviors toward her.

There is yet another issue. By definition, our patients are in a position of vulnerability. They come to us because they are struggling and looking for help. That puts us in a position of considerable power, that is, we have the power to influence whether their lives will proceed down a more satisfying and fulfilling path or a much more negative one. We have a special obligation to not take advantage of people in vulnerable positions, even if, on the surface, they agree to our proposals (APA Ethics Code, Principle E; CPA Code, I. Values Statement, II. Values Statement). Acting ethically in such a situation involves engaging in a complete and honest discussion regarding the services offered and careful questioning to make sure that the consent given, if that is the end result, is both fully informed and freely and willingly given. Learning how to reach the goal of a mutually acceptable outcome without any residual feelings of resentment or disappointment takes knowledge and the kind of skill that comes from careful and competent supervision.

The second primary ethical issue in this case concerns the involvement of Lynn's bank president. She or he encouraged Lynn's sister to refer Lynn for psychological treatment, and she or he subsequently requested updates from you regarding Lynn's condition and progress. Two issues are embedded in this aspect of the scenario: confidentiality, a complex issue we discuss first; and the professional role, which we discuss a bit later.

Keeping information we obtain from any source about people we work with professionally private is one of the most important values of our profession. Not only is keeping information private a crucial element of respect, but it also determines the degree of trust we receive, in both an individual and a broader perspective. If people tell us intimate and private things about their lives and learn that we have passed that information on, the chances of them telling us anything else of importance is near zero. In a broader sense, if the public at large does not have trust that psychologists will keep information confidential, they are not likely to seek out our services. Both the APA and the CPA codes speak repeatedly to this value (APA Ethics Code, Principle E, 1.04, 1.05, 1.06, 4.01, 4.04, 4.06, 4.07, 6.02, 8.05, 8.14, 8.15, 9.03; CPA Code, I. Values Statement, I.37–I.45, III.20) and again, the amount of attention given to this issue is reflective of its importance in our profession.

What should you do about Lynn's boss's request for information? Does the boss have a right to that information to determine whether Lynn can continue to work or, more magnanimously, to assist Lynn in being a good employee and thereby decreasing her anxiety about job security? In a word, no. The information Lynn provides you is private and no one has a right to that information—with five major exceptions.

The first exception involves *mandated reporting*, that is, situations in which you are required by law to report something that you learn during the course of providing a psychological service. These are those relatively extreme conditions in which the state (in the form of a legislature and a governor) have decided that public welfare or safety is more important than the general value of confidentiality in a professional relationship, so they have created a law that requires you to pass on information. Two such laws exist in many jurisdictions, although you will need to check the statutes and regulations in your own jurisdiction to know how these, or other situations, might apply. First, if you believe that Lynn is an imminent danger to an identified individual, you are often required to report that to the relevant authorities (e.g., police, family member, other persons who are in a position to prevent the dangerous behavior) as a means of protecting the potential victim despite the fact that taking such action violates the principle of confidentiality. This requirement is based on the well-known Tarasoff case that occurred in California in the 1970s, in which the California Supreme Court ruled that the mental health professionals involved in the treatment of their patient who made a threat against his former girlfriend have a duty to protect the potential victim. The majority opinion included the now famous statement, "The protective privilege ends where the public peril begins" (Tarasoff v. The Regents of the University of California, 1976). As a result, although the mental health professional has an obligation to protect the confidentiality of the patient, the California Court decided that there was a higher principle, and many state legislatures have subsequently developed statutes that clarify that the higher order obligation is to protect an identified victim from harm (Herbert & Young, 2002).

Be sure to check the laws and rules in your jurisdiction to determine whether such a report is required or only allowed. Different jurisdictions have used the Tarasoff ruling in different ways to write their laws, so they are not all the same (Herbert & Young, 2002). An allowed exception would mean that a law or rule permits you to release information, even if it does not require that you do so. That means that if you, in good faith (meaning that you have used adequate judgment and reasoning to draw your conclusion and you can present that reasoning to another professional in a reasonably convincing manner), report such a situation to proper authorities or individuals, you will not be accused or disciplined as a result of breaking confidentiality. The second type of report, this one mandated rather than merely allowed, is when you learn of a situation where a minor child or a vulnerable adult is being abused or neglected. You are then typically *required* to report that information to the appropriate state agency, typically a department of child protection, although the requirements differ substantially from jurisdiction to jurisdiction. From all of the information available to us at this point, these exceptions do not apply to Lynn.

The second general exception is a court order for release of private information. If you receive a court order for information, then you are required by law to release it. However, one can appear in front of a judge (or can appeal a judge's decision to a higher court) to argue that the information should be kept private and not revealed to anyone else, but the ruling of the judge (or appellate court) must be followed, if the psychologist wants to avoid legal consequences. If the request for information comes in the form of a subpoena it cannot be ignored, but a subpoena is not the same as a court order, unless the subpoena is signed by a judge. If a subpoena is received, a psychologist can request a hearing in front of a judge to hear arguments for why the subpoena should be quashed (withdrawn). You should carefully consult with your supervisor, and if needed, with an attorney knowledgeable about this type of law, if you receive a court order or subpoena to discuss its implications for your practice with the client, as well as your obligation to respond to them.

The third exception occurs when sharing the information you have is necessary to the services being offered. For example, your billing person has a right to have access to certain private information (not the entire file, but name, address, dates seen, etc.) to bill for your services. If you work in an organizational setting, other providers might have access to your file to provide comprehensive and competent services. For example, in hospitals, notes are often written in electronic charts to which many professionals might have access. Or you may work in a setting that has an on-call person for emergencies who has an ethical right to have access to your patients' files. In addition, you may be requested to submit information to the insurance company to meet their requirements for reimbursement of your services, if your patient has elected to use insurance coverage. This is a complex situation that requires a bit more consideration. If patients want to use their insurance to cover the cost of your services, it seems natural that these patients would expect you to comply with the release of information requirements of the insurance company to have their services covered. That may not always be the case, however, as some patients will not want any information released to their insurance company. When such a request occurs, it can be, at best, awkward for you, and even more than awkward if you have released information your patient wanted kept private. The best practice is to have every patient who desires to use insurance coverage sign a limited release of information form to allow you to share the information required by their insurance company. If they choose not to sign such a release, they always have the option of paying for your services privately.

The fourth exception occurs when a complaint is filed against you with a court or a licensing board. In such a circumstance, you may be compelled to release information in a patient record, for example, in the form of a subpoena from the board. Your patient could deny you permission to release those records. However, if you do not release the records to the board, you are subject to disciplinary action by the board for noncooperation with a board investigation. If at all possible, you want to avoid putting yourself in some disadvantageous position as a result of a choice made by your client. At the very least, you also deserve informed consent, that is, you should know in advance if you do not have permission to release records to a licensing board. However, we would never advise you to put yourself in that situation. If, in the unlikely event of a board complaint (less than 10% of psychologists have ever had a complaint filed against them; see Van Horne, 2004), you have a right to be able to take such action as is reasonably necessary to defend yourself. If your patient from the very beginning is unwilling to allow that, you should very seriously consider discontinuing the service. (It is not unethical for you to not provide a service.) It is only unethical to discriminate on the basis of legal categories, such as race, sexual orientation, or gender, or to abandon someone you are seeing, typically by not even providing the names of other professionals they can consult.

The fifth exception is when your patient gives you permission to share information with another individual or organization. For your self-protection (as well as to comply with laws or rules in many states or provinces), you should obtain this permission in writing. Similar to, but perhaps even more important than, the issue with informed consent for testing, the informed consent to release information should be undertaken with great care and with great respect and deference to the wishes of your patient. And it is important to remember that you are the professional, not your patient. Your patient may not have a clear understanding of what the consequences of releasing private information might be, so it is your responsibility to describe such potential consequences as part of the informed consent process. For instance in Lynn's case, if you release information to Lynn's boss, does Lynn's boss have a legal and ethical obligation to keep the information private? No. The boss may share the information with the human resources department, Lynn's direct supervisor, or others who the boss believes have a need to know. Information can travel quickly, particularly in this day and age. Lynn needs to understand that such sharing of information can occur before she can provide informed consent.

And, beyond the issue of informed consent to release information, an informed consent regarding the limits of confidentiality is needed. That is, as discussed above, your ability to keep information confidential is limited, that is, in cases of potential harm or if court ordered. Your patients do not have the knowledge you do about how therapy works and they have a right to know, from the very beginning, what those limitations are.

The second issue regarding the bank president has to do with the role you play in this scenario. You have been contacted to do an initial assessment, followed up with the provision of any psychological interventions that together you and Lynn decide might be of benefit to Lynn. Thus, you are primarily in the role of therapy provider. The assessment you conduct is going to have the goal of being helpful. Although objectivity and comprehensiveness are important in this context, both are of a different nature than if you were being hired to conduct a fitness for duty evaluation, a service that might have a major impact on Lynn's ability to maintain her employment and that might well end up in court, with you being called to testify as an expert witness. In providing therapy, the level of comprehensiveness of assessment may not be as great. In terms of the sources of information, the most important one will be what Lynn tells you. There may be some collateral information, what her sister reports initially, but there would usually not be an extended collateral interview. Likewise, some previous health records may be obtained, but likely not as many as would be obtained in a forensic assessment. How important are the psychological records for Lynn's treatment after her father's death 19 years ago? For most people, the event might be very important to explore, but the records from that time, less so. If a determination were made down the road that the records were important to obtain, Lynn would have to sign a release to acquire them. However, there would not be the presumption that they are important from the beginning, as they could be in a forensic assessment, for example.

Beyond the specific goals and sources of information involved in different forms of assessment, the role of therapist and the role of evaluator are quite different, and one moves from one into the other at some peril (S. Greenberg & Shuman, 1997, 2007; Strasburger, Gutheil, & Brodsky, 1997). Even if you are trying to be helpful to Lynn in communicating with the bank president, what if you provide information to Lynn's boss that he or she then uses to restrict Lynn's work or fire her? How is Lynn likely to feel about you in that case? That factor is apart from the fact that as a therapist, you are not in a position to make an objective assessment of how Lynn's progress relates to her ability to work. You should be focused primarily on how you can be helpful to Lynn, not on obtaining a comprehensive, objective assessment of Lynn's ability to work. Any attempt to do so opens the door to troubles for both you and Lynn. A very common complaint to licensing boards about psychologists has to do with exactly this kind of situation— a therapist attempting to provide input in a legal or employment context, believing that the input is objective. In fact, therapists often believe they have even better information because they have worked with the person for a period of time. What they fail to take into consideration is that the information they have is generally exclusively from the client. As such, it is neither totally objective nor verified. The rule in our opinion should be: Just don't do it.

Case 2—John Smith

The case of Mr. Smith raises a different, yet overlapping, set of ethical issues. It is important that this is primarily an assessment case, although it could potentially become a therapy case. The role of assessor is different from the role of therapist and raises a different set of ethical considerations. We consider here the following ethical issues in more detail: referral source expectations, competence, conflict of interest, informed consent, the advisability of collateral interviews, bias, and changing professional roles.

One of the first issues mentioned is that the cardiologist wants a report back on your work within 2 weeks. It is not unusual for a time frame to be provided in referrals, but such a time frame raises clinical, as well as ethical, concerns. Specifically, given that the primary goal of our work as mental health professionals is to provide competent services, What is the likelihood that a competent report can be generated within

2 weeks? That question becomes even more crucial when you discover that the exact referral question is absent and that the referring cardiologist is out of town and unable to provide additional guidance. The issues you would need to consider in determining whether you want to take on this referral have to do with your level of expertise and comfort with the specific type of referral, the accessibility of the data you will need to write a competent report, and the amount of time you have available. What if, for example, Mr. Smith is about to be discharged from the hospital and it turns out to be a week or more before you can see him? If the stars align just right, go for it! However, if there are reasons it might not be possible to do a competent job within 2 weeks, absolutely do not try to do it. Both authors of this text have seen licensed psychologists disciplined by licensing boards for taking on more than they should have and providing inadequate or harmful services, all with very good intentions.

The second, and perhaps most crucial, question always to ask yourself is, Do I have the competence to provide the psychological service being requested? In this case, it looks to be a situation of stress, perhaps depression and/or anxiety and/or a personality style prone to taking on too much, that has contributed to or is related to heart disease. Given that in the case scenario you did part of your postdoc in such a setting, you likely are competent, but if you are not (and here, being brutally honest with yourself is not only important but also sometimes career saving), the appropriate action would be to decline the referral or immediately seek out supervision/consultation from a psychologist with more expertise in the area than you. The case does specify that you have not worked with an individual with the diagnosis unstable angina (I20.0) before. A specific medical diagnosis is not likely to rule out competence for you, if you have dealt with similar cases (i.e., cases with similar psychological issues), although differing ICD–10–CM diagnoses may well rule out competence for you if you have not received training and supervision in providing clinical services to people with a specific set of problems in the past. However, there is always a consideration regarding competence that you should think about, as every individual is different. The APA Ethics Code does not (and should not) require that you get supervision or consultation with every single person you see because that person is, by definition, going to be different from everyone else you have seen (see Bersoff, 2008; Fisher, 2003; Sommers-Flanagan & Sommers-Flanagan, 2007). But not only is competence an important issue to ensure that you first, do no harm but it is also one of the primary reasons for disciplinary action by licensing boards (Association of State and Provincial Psychology Boards, 2014b; Rodolfa et al., 2013). So, it behooves you to be honest with yourself about your level of competence before taking on a professional situation that is in any way new for you without seeking supervision/consultation as part of the services you offer. In this case, let us assume that you are competent, so you decide to proceed.

The third issue involves your review of the hospital chart, which indicates that part of the problem may be job-related stress (at this point this is a hypothesis to be tested through gathering additional data). Because you know someone well who works at the same place, you have to decide whether it is a good idea for you to work with Mr. Smith. The first of two questions to answer is, Does your contact with Mark (your significant other's brother) present a conflict of interest that might make it difficult for you to be open and objective in working with Mr. Smith? Do you know something about the workplace (either positive or negative) that already leads you to think in some specific way about Mr. Smith? If any part of the answer to that question is a yes, then you should not accept the referral, responding to Dr. Jones that a personal conflict of interest prevents you from working with Mr. Smith. Even if in your honest assessment of the situation you decide that you can be completely unbiased and objective, you should ask yourself whether it is possible that you might find out information about the company or about Mark that you would prefer not to know. For example, what if you found out that racial discrimination were part of the stress Mr. Smith experiences, and further, you find out that Mark is one of the people causing that stress? Would knowing that have the potential for causing problems in your relationship with your significant other? Again, if the answer in any way is yes, or could be yes, it is better to communicate to Dr. Jones (even with the time deadline) that you are not able to accept the referral because of a personal conflict of interest. As a student (or newly licensed psychologist), you may be very curious and inclined to take on this likely very interesting case. You will reach a point in your career, either by taking the advice of others or through a negative experience of your own, that you will undoubtedly realize it is better to avoid problems before they develop. Hopefully, you already know this and do not need to learn it through negative experiences in the future.

An important issue raised by this case has to do with informed consent, a slightly different aspect of informed consent issues with Lynn. As indicated in Chapter 5 when you are working in an outpatient setting and someone seeks your service, it is reasonable to assume that they are coming to you voluntarily and that they know what you do and something of the purpose of the session. There certainly are circumstances in which that is not the case, such as a court-ordered referral. Such forensic referrals raise a whole other list of issues to consider (see S. Greenberg & Shuman, 1997, 2007) that are beyond the scope of this text.

In an inpatient medical setting, one should not make an assumption of informed consent. It is possible that the referring physician has

made a decision that your services might be helpful without so informing the patient. Or, at least, you should not assume that such a conversation occurred between the physician and the patient. Therefore, it is
ethically incumbent on you to spend sufficient time determining what
the patient's starting point is. Typically, starting with something along
the lines of the following can be helpful: "Dr. Jones referred you to see
me and I'm wondering whether you and Dr. Jones had a conversation about that and what your thoughts are about working with me."
Beyond that, it will be important for you to explain who you are, what
you do, and something of what your goals are, in this case, determining what Mr. Smith's experiences and needs might be. It is perfectly
appropriate to say that you have very little information about him, so
you need to learn more about him and why he is in the hospital and
why Dr. Jones has referred him to you. Even before you start asking
questions, however, you ought to find out whether Mr. Smith has any
questions of you that you can answer. This same point can and should
be made with every patient you see. He may well have questions that
have to do with whether you are a person who will likely be able to
relate to him and understand him. Although that may (or may not) be
an issue in this case because of ethnic, age, or gender differences, the
question about whether you can relate is one that every single patient
you see is likely to have, regardless of how similar or different in background and experience you are to that person. Patients are expected
to reveal, in a very honest manner, very personal and private aspects
of themselves. Without such honesty, we have limited or skewed data
on which to make decisions or recommendations. But, of course, they
are going to wonder whether you are a person who is trustworthy and
sensitive enough for them to do so with you. Your job will be to demonstrate, in small, but consistent, behavioral ways over time that you
are exactly that kind of person, recognizing that trust gets built slowly
over time but can be broken down very quickly.

So, Mr. Smith could ask questions about your vocational history,
your experience in dealing with medical patients, your family circumstances, your experience in dealing with people of different ethnic backgrounds from yourself (for those of you who are from a different ethnic
background from Mr. Smith). Because of theoretical and personality differences, mental health professionals may differ in the degree to which
they are willing to answer those questions directly and completely. We
believe that honest sharing of yourself, with limits on how personal the
information is that you share, is one way of communicating that this
professional relationship is one in which directness and self-disclosure
is expected and respected (see Derlega & Berg, 1987; Farber, 2006; Lee,
2014). It is sometimes useful to ask yourself before responding to a specific question, Would I be willing in a different context to tell someone

the same information about myself? Or, more important, Can I imagine a scenario in which I might later feel uncomfortable in answering this question directly? If the answer to this second question could be yes, trust your own reactions, and rather than answering the question, ask the person why knowing that would be helpful to him/her.

Last, with regard to informed consent, you need to make clear to Mr. Smith that he can decide not to talk with you and that there will be no negative consequences from you. Further, you need to let Mr. Smith know that you will communicate to Dr. Jones that your work together was discussed and Mr. Smith decided that it would not be in his best interest to continue the professional relationship; that is, he needs to know that you will report his decision in an objective manner, such that Dr. Jones would be unlikely to draw negative conclusions about him as a result.

We discussed collateral interviews briefly in Chapter 3. At times, getting the input of another individual might be helpful—especially when the patient is a child and the collateral source is a parent or, sometimes, a teacher. Custodial parents have a legal right to know when health services are being provided to their children, so there are no legal concerns regarding confidentiality in talking with them, although there may be clinical concerns in discussing your work with a child with his/her parents, as children often desire confidentiality, even from their parents (Sattler & Schaffer, 2014), but that is an issue beyond the scope of this text. With adults, however, a collateral interview, by definition, means a violation of confidentiality. In some circumstances, the patient desires such collateral contact and gives permission for you to talk to someone else. That can happen with the patient being unaware of all of the potential consequences of such collateral contact. It is your task as the professional to understand what the various consequences could be and to have a thorough informed consent conversation before making any contact with collateral sources. The other variable to weigh is what the potential benefits, as well as the expected benefits, might be. Just because there is a significant other (whether a family member or colleague or employer) does not mean that you should seek permission to contact that person. You should have a good idea of what information you are looking for, who might be able to provide that information, and how it relates to either the assessment or the intervention process before you proceed with the informed consent discussion with your patient. Most often, in reality, collateral interviews would not be conducted in this type of situation, for two reasons. Conducting such interviews often provides only limited additional clinical information, and it is often not worth the extra cost to undertake. You should have a good idea of what information you are looking for and who might be able to provide that information and how that information relates to either the assessment or the intervention process before you proceed with the informed consent discussion with your patient.

Even more important are confidentiality issues. In a clinical situation, contacting his employer or his colleagues by definition reveals that Mr. Smith has psychological issues that warrant the involvement of a psychologist. Even if Mr. Smith gives his permission, breaking that confidentiality might not be worth the amount of additional information obtained.

Mr. Smith is in a committed and satisfactory gay relationship. That may raise moral concerns for you, depending on your own background. The APA and CPA ethical codes make clear that it is unethical to discriminate against people because of their sexual orientation, and federal law makes it clear that it is illegal to do so. If you are a person who cannot be objective and unbiased because of Mr. Smith's sexual orientation, then you should not work with him, and a referral is appropriate. In making the referral, however, it is ethically essential that you not communicate or imply in any way that you're not working with him is a result of some deficit, lack, or inappropriateness in him. You need to own and take responsibility for your own views.

The last ethical issue raised by this case has to do with changing roles. You were asked to conduct a psychological assessment to assist the physician in knowing how to proceed, likely including knowing whether a referral for psychotherapy would be helpful. Assuming you do psychotherapy, should you take on such a referral after you have conducted the assessment? Such a change in roles is rarely advisable in certain circumstances, such as conducting an assessment for forensic purposes after having provided treatment (see S. Greenberg & Shuman, 2007). Going from having provided an assessment to providing treatment is more nuanced. A number of questions need to be considered.

First and foremost is the question, Is there something about the nature of the assessment, the nature of the professional relationship that has developed, or the individual you assessed that would make it difficult for that person to be able to manage a shift in roles comfortably and without confusion? This question has both to do with your relationship with Mr. Smith and Mr. Smith's relationship with you. Has a relationship developed that would be hard to translate into a supportive therapeutic one? Mr. Smith's having been somewhat guarded in his responses, perhaps out of fear of how the assessment might impact his life, would be one such example. Or perhaps he told you more than he later felt comfortable doing, and that would make continued therapeutic contact difficult.

Second, might there be a need for a follow-up, formal assessment at some point that will make your taking on the whole range of psychological services confusing or disadvantageous to being helpful? That is, if the assessment process has gone well and you have developed a good working relationship with Mr. Smith, then if there is a need for a follow-up assessment, you would be the appropriate person to undertake that psychological service. However, if, in the meantime, you have switched roles from assessor to therapist, going back to being an assessor is fraught with complications (see Greenberg & Shuman, 2007).

Third, might your approach to doing the initial assessment be influenced by the prospect of providing therapy after the assessment has been concluded? That is, might you be biased in the sense that you would be more inclined to conclude there are problems present for which therapy would be helpful, if you had in mind that you might be able to provide that therapy, whether that is because you want the experience, as a trainee or newly licensed psychologist, or because you want the additional income from providing what could be long-term therapy? If the answer to any of these questions is yes, you should keep these roles clearly separate.

Case 3—Anne Sanchez

The case of Ms. Sanchez is different from the first two cases in that it is strictly an assessment case, and the probability of it being a forensic case is fairly high. That is, it is likely that your report will be used by the referring attorney as part of a case she or he makes for federal income support, especially if your report is favorable to Ms. Sanchez's potential legal case, which immediately raises a question for you of role and objectivity. If there is pressure from the attorney or from Ms. Sanchez, even subtle pressure in the sense that you come to like her and want to be helpful to her, can you remain objective in your role as an independent evaluator, rather than coloring your findings to fit your hopes to be helpful? That is a dilemma that every psychologist who does assessments faces with virtually every case. It takes a good deal of self-awareness and honesty with oneself, as well as a thorough understanding of the APA Ethics Code Standard 3.05 (a)(1) (APA, 2010), to remain within an acceptable range of objectivity.

The probability is also well above zero that you could be called to testify. Most cases settle before going to court, but if you do this kind of work, sooner or later you will be called to testify, both in a deposition and live in court. This raises the question of competence: Do you have experience and training in providing forensic services? Forensic psychology is a specialty area unto itself and requires a considerable amount of knowledge, skill, and supervised experience, not only about a specific type of assessment but also about the law, to provide forensic services competently. If you have such competence, proceed. If you do not, either decline the referral or seek consultation with the goal of learning a new area of practice (APA Ethics Code, Standard 2.01c; CPA Code, Ethical Standard II.8). Note the language in the APA (2010) Standard 2.01c about what is necessary to become competent in a new area: "Psychologists planning to provide services, teach, or conduct research involving populations, areas, techniques, or technologies new to them undertake relevant education, training, supervised experience, consultation, or study" (p. 5).

Conducting a psychological assessment raises a number of ethical issues, some of which have not yet been fully considered in this chapter. First, are the data-gathering methods used appropriate to the case? This means are the tests and methods used current (the latest version with validity data appropriate to current use) and consistent with the psychological literature, and are the tests and methods valid for the purposes being used (APA Ethics Code, Standard 9.02; CPA Code Ethical Standard II.21)? These issues were discussed earlier, specifically when examining the specific psychological tests with the case of Lynn.

In addition, the case description states that Ms. Sanchez is Mexican American. Does that mean that Spanish is her first language? If yes, how fluent is she in English? Even if fluent, is she more comfortable in Spanish and should Spanish tests be used? Are you fluent in Spanish, or if English is the appropriate language, do you have sufficient background in understanding and working with Mexicans or Mexican Americans that you can do so competently (APA, 1990, 2010)? Ethnic and language backgrounds can influence results on psychological tests and in assessment behaviors more generally in a host of ways (APA, 1990, 2002b).

Second, are the methods being used to gather information sufficient to answer the referral question or questions (APA Ethics Code, Standard 9.01; CPA Code Ethical Standard II.13)? The types of testing needed and the degree to which the tests chosen are adequate are discussed in Chapter 6 (this volume). So, this issue is both an ethical and a clinical question.

Third, does the written report adequately document the procedures used, the bases for any conclusions drawn or recommendations made, and any limitations of the conclusions and recommendations, based on the availability of data, the limitations of the tests used, or the level of involvement by the client in the assessment process (APA Ethics Code, Standard 9.01; CPA Code, Ethical Standards II.21 and III.8)? Here, it is also important to be honest with oneself. As stated in Chapter 2 (this volume), as human beings, we are quite capable of convincing ourselves that our opinions have validity even when they do not. Being clear not only about the limitations in general of what we do as psychologists but also about the specific limitations inherent in our tests or other methods is an absolute requirement of competent and ethical practice. Every psychological evaluation report should have a paragraph including the limitations of the assessment, because every psychological assessment has limitations. Nearly every psychological assessment also has conflicting evidence, where one source of information suggests one conclusion and another source, a different conclusion. It is important to include a discussion of those differences and to provide a rationale for why one set of data is given preference over the other in reaching the ultimate conclusions.

All evaluees have an ethical right to receive feedback on the results of the testing (APA Ethics Code, Standard 9.10; CPA Code, Ethical Standard III.15). Whether patients want or seek out feedback or not might be a function of many factors, including the setting of the service offered. In the experience of one of the authors of this text, having completed a few thousand assessments during his career, it is not unusual for patients not to seek feedback sessions. The point, however, is that you have an ethical obligation to offer and provide feedback if the patient would like to hear your evaluation. In fact, some patients will actively seek feedback, and when you provide them this session, it is wise to think about feedback as a process of two-way communication (Finn, 1996; Fischer, 2000; Levak, Siegel, Nichols, & Stolberg, 2011). You will be providing information, but you will also be receiving considerable information in the form of the person's reactions to your information. Take note; those reactions could be valuable in your understanding of the person. It is best to start with questions regarding the person's goals and concerns for the session and focus much of what you say on those issues. It usually works best to pick a limited number of major interpretations, rather than trying to cover everything. Doing the latter will likely only confuse or overwhelm the person. Pick those interpretations or conclusions that are most related to the stated goals of the person. Avoid psychological jargon as much as possible. The goal is to provide feedback that will be understandable and useful to the person, not to impress him or her with your knowledge or command of the material. It typically works best to start with information that is consistent with the person's beliefs about himself or herself, then to add information that might be new, and last to provide conclusions that could be threatening to the person's self-concept or self-esteem or difficult for the person to hear. If the person perceives your feedback in that way, she or he may reject your interpretations. If you experience resistance, do not try to convince the person that you are right. Start by listening. It is useful to ask if there is anything in the interpretation that does seem correct. But, it is also perfectly acceptable in the face of ongoing resistance to say, "Well, that is what the test indicated, but sometimes our tests are wrong." It is acceptable to say this, because it is a very true statement!

For many tests, including the MMPI–2, computerized interpretations can be obtained. Be cautious about their use (APA Ethics Code, Standard 9.06). Although they can provide helpful language to use in your report, they are typically based on a prototypical profile. Virtually every real-life profile will have differences from the prototypical profile, which will result in different characteristics or problems. It is your job to interpret the tests, not simply to rely on a computerized interpretation. Both authors of this text have seen cases in which psychologists have been disciplined by licensing boards for using computerized reports verbatim in their reports without attribution of the source and for using language from a computerized report that did not fit the overall data from the testing of the person. This is another situation where the adage "just don't do it" might apply.

In broader terms, what we are suggesting with our use of the language "just don't do it" is that you develop practice habits early in your career that are based on a sound ethical foundation, on developing competence, and on good risk management practices (see Chapter 8). For a discussion of the neuroscience of habits and why they can be difficult to change once developed, see Graybiel and Smith (2014).

Now we come to a part of this case that is critical in the practice of psychology: response to a flirtatious or sexualized interaction with a client (see Barnett, 2014). You have noticed that Ms. Sanchez acted in a sexualized manner, including provocative dress and flirtatious behaviors. What is the appropriate response on your part? The only part of the answer to that question that is easy and unambiguous is that you do not, under any circumstances, react in a parallel sexualized manner (APA Ethics Code, Standard 10.05; CPA Code, Ethical Standard II, 27). What do you do, then? The very first thing you should think about is consultation with trusted colleagues. In this case description, you as the psychologist are lucky to have two colleagues with whom you meet regularly—Use them! Your discussion with them should include a description of Ms. Sanchez's behavior, including its frequency, intensity, and consistency over time, as well as an honest description of what your reactions, all of them, were. The discussion should include a consideration of the potential meaning and purpose of her behavior; what your reactions mean; and in particular, a consideration of whether you can work with her in an objective, unbiased manner.

Beyond the general recommendation of consultation, one question that will be helpful in deciding what to do is to ask yourself what meaning her behavior might have. Does her behavior have a purpose? For example, is she trying to gain your favor and simply has a limited repertoire of behavior to choose from, with sexualized behaviors being one form of interaction with which she has experience? Is she lonely, such that it is a more social act than meaningful in the context of the professional interaction? Is it more blatantly an attempt at a bribe to cause you to write a report that will be helpful to her? Is she intellectually capable of devising such a scheme? Is it possible that it is a strategy devised by her attorney? Or by someone else close to her? Does she seem to be aware of her own behavior or does she seem oblivious? The answers to those questions could provide you with valuable insight into her psychological and intellectual functioning, so the behavior has importance beyond the impact that it has or might have on you. That impact also plays a role, however. What is your reaction? Do you find her behavior attractive? Does it confuse you? Does it repulse you? Do you feel manipulated? Does it make you feel attractive? Is it distracting to you? Is it hard to concentrate on the verbal information she is providing you?

What you decide to do will depend in part on the answers to some or all of these questions. You should thoroughly discuss any of the questions that are relevant with your colleagues, or if it occurs while you are a student, with a supervisor. If the behavior is distracting or affects your concentration, you need to tell the patient that and ask her to stop. If her behavior is such, or your reactions are such, that you feel some risk of crossing a boundary, or if you believe her behavior might escalate such that you will have a more difficult situation to deal with later, you need to be very clear with her about boundaries and about your lack of tolerance for any attempts on her part to cross boundaries. Mind you, "lack of tolerance" does not mean intolerance, that is, punishing or striking back at her in some way. It means merely that you will not accept nor respond to such boundary crossings. Asking her to stop can be done gently and with sensitivity, such that she might change her behavior with very little negative impact on your professional relationship and little emotional reactivity on her part. At most, it might result in a bit of embarrassment. The second response, directly confronting her behavior, is much more likely to impact her feelings about you and the assessment process, perhaps undermining trust and making it difficult to continue the assessment. That is not to say that is an inappropriate response. If her behavior is clearly seductive in nature and continues despite your lack of response, then such a response might be necessary. However, it is not without risks.

A third type of response on your part might be to do nothing overtly. Certainly, your covert behaviors would all have to do with not reacting to her actions. But if her behaviors are not too blatant or overt or continuous and you are not distracted by them, noting them as you do any other of her behaviors and including them in your psychological interpretations of her might be the most appropriate response. Refraining from responding in an overt way has the lowest level of risk to the professional relationship (assuming that her flirtations do not tempt you) and maximizes the probability that you will be able to continue to conduct an objective assessment of her. The two deciding points about whether such a reaction could work, both clinically and ethically, will likely be how direct and continuous her sexual behaviors are, on the one hand, and what the nature of your internal reactions are, on the other. If both are below some reasonable threshold, such that an appropriately professional and objective relationship can continue, then that might be the best option. This is another point at which unsparing honesty with oneself, as well as consultation with one's peers or supervisors, is critical.

Clearly, ethics is a critical and complicated issue in the practice of psychology. Our intent here has been to demonstrate, in the context of specific cases, how ethical issues occur constantly and due consideration of them is essential (see also Nagy, 2005, 2011). Our hope is that you will avail yourself of the knowledge and expertise of your faculty, supervisors, and, eventually, consultants, as you struggle, to use the language of Plato, to do the right thing.

Risk Management—Protecting Your Patients and Yourself

8

R isk management is a process designed to minimize negative events and outcomes and to maximize positive events and outcomes for both the psychologist and the patient. It involves identifying what could go wrong and developing an intentional plan of action to deal with the risks inherent in the situation in the most effective manner possible. Ethical considerations are primarily concerned with the well-being of the patient, although risk management involves the well-being of both the patient and the psychologist. In cases of an obvious incompatibility of positive outcomes or avoidance of negative outcomes for both psychologist and patient, the patient's needs and goals remain primary. However, nothing is unethical or unprofessional per se in the psychologist taking reasonable steps to protect himself or herself from negative outcomes. In summary, *risk management* is the process by which psychologists attempt to decrease negative outcomes to themselves while also keeping the patient's well-being fully in mind. We see the concept of risk management as something similar to a

http://dx.doi.org/10.1037/14778-009
A Student's Guide to Assessment and Diagnosis Using the ICD–10–CM: Psychological and Behavioral Conditions, by J. Schaffer and E. Rodolfa

stool with four legs: (a) professional relationship, (b) ethical practice, (c) competence, and (d) consideration of professional threats.

None of us psychologists are perfect and all of us will make mistakes, some of which could be the occasion for a letter of complaint to a licensing board or a malpractice lawsuit. Although neither of the authors has been sued or had a complaint filed with a licensing board, as licensing board members, we have participated in the adjudication of many complaints. On the basis of this experience, we firmly believe that one way to minimize the possibility of such an event is to have positive professional relationships with your clients. Such relationships do not occur spontaneously; they occur because the psychologist treats the patient with respect, exhibits concern about the patient's well-being, and responds to the patient's concerns. In essence, the psychologist uses clinical competencies to develop and maintain positive relationship with patients.

Among the most helpful perspectives regarding the development of such relationships came from Carl Rogers, with subsequent work by Charles Truax and Robert Carkhuff (1967, 2007; Carkhuff, 2009), suggesting that there are three central relationship factors: congruence, empathy, and unconditional positive regard. Clients tend to be quite forgiving when they feel respected, cared for, and understood. If you feel tension or conflict in the relationship, or a therapeutic rupture occurs, take heed and use your clinical skills to do what you can to repair the rupture (Horvath & Bedi, 2002; Safran, Crocker, McMain, & Murray, 1990).

As you develop relationships through the display of empathy, unconditional positive regard and congruence, it is critical that you meet patients where they are. As each of your patients will be diverse, they will all be different from you, although they will have aspects of their personhood that are more or less similar and familiar to your own. Many factors may make a client similar to or different from you (Sue & Torino, 2005), including ethnic group, social class, gender, gender orientation, and religion, as well as his or her own histories of experience. These complexities can feel overwhelming, but remember many resources can help you assess and treat your diverse patients. For instance, Cornish, Schreier, Nadkarni, Metzger, and Rodolfa (2010) created a text with specific suggestions and guidelines to treat the increasingly diverse population in our country. Bhui and Morgan (2007) provided an overview of "culturally capable practice" that encourages practitioners to (a) understand their views of race and ethnicity; (b) understand how differences in views of mental health, family, and community and differences in communication behaviors can affect practice; and (c) discuss similarities and differences when needed. Guidelines from the American Psychological Association (APA) and many books provide practitioners summaries of the issues involved in treating an increasingly diverse population (see Chapter 10, this volume). Thus, in addition to empathy, positive regard, and congruence, a multiculturally capable mental health practitioner will build strong clinical relationships by being sensitive not only to who his or her patients are but also how he or she reacts to and feels about them. In other words, self-reflexive practice is essential.

The second important aspect of protecting yourself from adverse outcomes is to practice ethically, the second leg of the stool, which also means practicing within the boundaries of your areas of competence, the third leg. Do not, we repeat, do not try to do more than your role and skills as psychologist allow you to do. We have reviewed board complaints where psychologists got into trouble because they tried to do more than they were competent to do and thereby overstepped the boundaries of ethical practice. Typically, these psychologists did not have exploitative or self-aggrandizing intent but rather lacked an adequate ethical foundation for their actions. Practicing competently and in accordance with ethical standards, and developing effective professional relationships, go a long way toward decreasing the risks involved in the practice of psychology.

The fourth leg of our stool is careful consideration of the possible professional threats that may occur when working with each person/group/ organization. That is, what could possibly go wrong? In a word, lots. Therefore, having considered at some length elsewhere in this text the first three legs of our stool (see, e.g., the Introduction and Chapters 2 and 7, this volume), in this chapter, we spend time considering the fourth, professional threats.

A first consideration that covers all professional activities has to do with the policies you have that govern your practice. Four issues are particularly important to your practice each and every day, and as a result, you should know and understand each of them. They are

(a) the laws and rules that govern the practice of psychology in your jurisdiction,
(b) the federal Health Insurance Portability and Accountability Act (HIPAA, 1996; see U.S. Department of Health and Human Services, 2015),
(c) informed consent, and
(d) release of information.

Laws and Rules

Three categories of guiding principles govern the practice of psychology in each jurisdiction. First are the statutes passed by state, provincial, or territorial legislatures that place in law the requirements and boundaries for professional practice. Taken as a totality, such statutes are usually referred to as the *Practice Act.* Most Practice Acts have a section that says something like, "The Board may [or shall] adopt such rules as are necessary to carry out the provisions of this Act." Thus, most licensing boards also develop a set of rules (also referred to as *regulations*) that define the basis for licensure, specifications of continuing education, and the definition of practice conduct (i.e., rules of conduct) that constitute minimum acceptable practice and the violation of which can lead to disciplinary action. It is essential that every practicing psychologist knows and understands the laws and rules that govern the practice of psychology in his or her jurisdiction. That is the minimum level of ethical and legal conduct to which the state (in the form of the licensing board) can hold a licensee accountable and that can result in disciplinary action that affects the right to practice.

Although reviewing the rules of the 64 jurisdictions in the United States and Canada seemed like an impossibly daunting task that would only lead to a confusing amount of potentially contradictory information, the Association of State and Provincial Psychology Boards (ASPPB), the association composed of the licensing boards in the United States and Canada, has model language regarding providing psychological assessments that serves as a model for many jurisdictional rules in this area. These model (ASPPB, 2002) regulations make the following points:

- Psychologists should not offer a professional opinion about someone without substantial professional contact or a formal assessment of that person.
- Information obtained in the course of an assessment should be considered confidential.
- Patients have a right to obtain an explanation of the assessment procedures and of the results of the assessment in language they can reasonably be expected to understand.
- In formal psychological reports psychologists state any reservations they have regarding conclusions, limitations of the assessment procedures, any conflicting information present in the assessment data, and the use of any nonstandard assessment procedures.
- In their communications with nonpsychologists, psychologists are careful not to reveal information, such as test questions or answers, that would compromise the fairness, objectivity, or integrity of the psychological testing process.
- The publication of any testing materials by a psychologist shall be accompanied by material that describes the rationale for and development of the test, evidence for its reliability and validity, and the characteristics of the normative sample. The specific purposes and intended contexts for the tests uses should be clearly described.

There is a third category related to laws and rules that is more difficult to track, because it falls more within the practice of law than the practice of psychology, yet it is important that every psychologist have an awareness of the requirements that this category may place on professional practice. Any psychologist can challenge the existence of any law or rule, but such challenge can only come in the form of a challenge to an action of a licensing board or the decision of a court. The legal title for such a challenge is an *appeal*. An appeal of the decision of a licensing board usually goes to a district court. An appeal of the decision of a district court goes to an appellate court. An appeal of the decision of an appellate court goes to the supreme court. Most often, although not always, an appellate or supreme court will publish a written opinion that offers a basis for the decision reached. Such a written opinion, referred to as *case law*, unlike the rulings of a licensing board or a district court, become precedent for future cases, that is, they take on the force of law in the geographic jurisdiction of the court. Thus, if there is case law in a particular area of practice, a psychologist may be bound to practice within the framework defined by that case law.

HIPAA

The second legal requirement involves compliance with HIPAA, which covers the practice of psychology throughout the United States. HIPAA is a federal law with multifaceted goals, one of which was designed to address privacy by defining consistent standards across all jurisdictions throughout the United States regarding electronic communication for insurance claims. Perhaps the most important goal of HIPAA was describing the requirements to protect the privacy of patient's personal health information. The three primary aspects of HIPAA's requirements for health practitioners are (a) the Privacy Rule, (b) the Security Rule, and (c) the Transaction Rule.

THE PRIVACY RULE

The Privacy Rule establishes the minimum requirements for all health professionals, including psychologists, for disclosing private information of a patient. This rule describes the circumstances when you can release patient information, and when patient consent is and is not required to disclose such information. The Privacy Rule requires that patients receive a statement from the practitioner of the limits of the privacy of their personal health information. In addition, the Privacy Rule provides patients the right to (a) receive notice when their records will be released, (b) within limits access their health record, and (c) modify their health record (APA Practice Organization, n.d.). Figure B.1 in Appendix B provides an example of a Privacy Practices statement required by the Privacy Rule.

THE SECURITY RULE

The Security Rule, the second component of HIPAA, "outlines the steps a psychologist must take to protect confidential information from *unintended* disclosure through breaches of security" (APA Practice Organization, n.d.). The Security Rule requires that a psychologist and other health care professionals maintain the security, confidentiality, integrity, and availability of electronic personal health information. To meet the standards of the Security Rule, the psychologist should begin with an analysis of their electronic practices. As guidance, the Security Rule has three standards that specify minimum requirements for the Rule's implementation. Administrative standards describe how policies and procedures, including staff training, should be implemented to secure electronic personal health information. Physical standards emphasize the security of the physical space where the computer server containing the electronic health information is stored, such as appropriate locks. Technical standards focus on the transmission and authentication issues that may emerge when electronic personal health information is accessed. Thus, for example, technical standards involve the development of policies and procedures regarding who has access to a patient's electronic personal health information or how the computer system will be monitored for security breaches.

Because the practice of psychology for each psychologist is unique, the Security Rule can be complied with in various ways. Thus, we strongly recommend accessing the APA Practice Organization (n.d.) resources or the U.S. Department of Health and Human Services website (http://www.hhs.gov/ocr/privacy/hipaa/administrative/securityrule) for guidance.

THE TRANSACTION RULE

The Transaction Rule considers the technical aspects of transmitting an electronic message containing electronic health care information. Thus, if a psychologist were to send electronic personal health care information to an insurance company, the sender and recipient would have to comply with the rules set forth in the Transaction Rule. The technical nature of this Rule is beyond the scope of this book, so we encourage you to seek resources to learn more about this Rule and HIPAA in general. Information about the Transaction rule can be downloaded from the U.S. Department of Health and Human Services website at http://www.cms. gov/Regulations-and-Guidance/HIPAA-Administrative-Simplification/ TransactionCodeSetsStands/Downloads/txfinal.pdf.

As you can see, HIPAA is a complex series of laws and regulations. This brief discussion provides you an overview of its essential features. As a student of psychology, you should understand that HIPAA provides a floor for minimal requirements to practice, and if state requirements are more demanding regarding patient privacy, the likelihood is that you will need to follow the most stringent laws and regulations.

For more information, however, multiple resources are available to provide you additional helpful information, including books and websites. Two websites that are particularly useful are the HIPAA site of the U.S. Department of Health and Human Services (http://www.hhs.gov/ocr/privacy/) and the website developed by APA for its practitioner members (http://www.apapracticecentral.org/business/hipaa/index.aspx). These two sites provide additional information about the privacy and security rules and an overview of a psychologist's obligations under HIPAA. For the present, if you have questions about HIPAA requirements, seek advice and consultation from your supervisor, an attorney, or an expert who understand the complex rules and regulations of HIPAA.

Informed Consent

The second policy/document that you should carefully consider is an informed consent form. You will want your patients to sign this, but it is first and foremost a process that includes informing your patients, in clear, understandable language, who you are and what you intend to do, along with all of the reasonably conceivable consequences of the psychological service you are proposing, so that the patient or patients can freely and intentionally decide whether they want to continue their professional relationship with you or not. Thus, informed consent is not only a legal issue, it is also an ethical issue. Respecting the autonomy (APA, 2010) and the dignity of persons (Canadian Psychological Association [CPA], 2000) is a fundamental ethical principle in both the APA and CPA codes of ethics.

Despite its importance, informed consent is often not given adequate consideration. For example, Krumholz (2010) found that the procedures to inform patients through the use of 540 informed consent forms in 157 hospitals were inadequate. Pope and Vasquez (2011) succinctly described the importance of the informed consent process as follows:

> This fundamental concept can trip us up if we are not careful. Nothing blocks a patient's access to help with such cruel efficiency as a bungled attempt at informed consent. . . . The doors to our offices and clinics are wide open. The resources are all in place. But not even the most persistent patients can make their way past intimidating forms (which clerks may shove at patients

when they first arrive), our set speeches full of noninformative information, and our nervous attempts to meet externally imposed legalistic requirements such as the Health Insurance Portability and Accountability Act. A first step is to recognize that informed consent is not a static ritual but a useful process. (p. 171)

Cressey (2012) reported that after receiving informed consent, 70% of 200 patients in the study did not understand that they were receiving unproven treatments. Cressey recommended that the informed consent process be based on interactive forms and procedures to better inform patients.

We agree. We believe that this potentially automatic process can be performed efficiently and effectively. To do so, we have provided a generic form as an example and, more importantly, a list of factors that are important to include in the informed consent process, or at least minimally should be considered as you seek to inform your patients of the critical issues related to their assessment and treatment.

In Figure B.2 in Appendix B, we have provided a generic version of an agency informed consent form. We believe, however, it is necessary to provide this caveat: Do not use this form as is, rather this generic form should be revised to include specific jurisdictional (i.e., state, province, territory) requirements, given that each jurisdiction has its own laws and regulations.

As you develop an informed consent form to fit your setting and develop a process to discuss the informed consent issues, it will be helpful for you to seek supervision and consult carefully about what the jurisdictional and ethical requirements are. For the purposes of this text, we believe it is critical to provide you the following list of factors that should be considered and likely should be included in any informed consent process (note not just included in the form).

1. A description of what your training and background is that gives you the competence to provide the proposed services. This could be in the form of a brief description in an informed consent form or it could be in a separate document that describes you and your practice.

2. Which specific services you are proposing and the basis for those services, based on your assessment of the person/situation and the appropriate diagnostic category from the Clinical Modification of the *International Statistical Classification of Diseases and Related Health Problems* (ICD–10–CM; National Center for Health Statistics, 2015). Obviously, the rationale for your services is something that changes over time. It is best to acquire some degree of informed consent from the very first session, but you may not yet know exactly what your proposed treatment will be until you have gathered more information. For example, you may well decide which psychological tests to use or whether

to obtain collateral information only after the interview, which you will use as a basis for deciding what other sources of information you need. And you cannot decide on the ICD–10–CM diagnosis that will serve as a basis for your proposed services until you have sufficient information. The important point is that informed consent is an ongoing process. It is not something that is obtained at the beginning of the relationship and then lasts for all time. It is something that should be reviewed anytime there are any changes in perspective, diagnosis, direction, goals, or proposed psychological services.

3. A list of alternative services (including therapy, assessment, consultation, or supervision) that might be used to address the same set of problems and why you have chosen the approaches you have. This is obviously a somewhat gray area. Given the amount of research that has accumulated over the past 40-plus years (see Bergin & Garfield, 1971; Hunsley & Lee, 2014; Lambert, 2013), it would not be possible to provide all of the alternatives for which there is empirical support. To attempt to do so would be overwhelming to your patients and would violate the first principle of true informed consent, providing information that is understandable and on which the person can make a free and informed choice. What is appropriate to provide is a limited number of reasonable options, so the patient can know that there are viable alternatives from which to choose.

4. A description of the limitations and potentially negative outcomes of your proposed services. This is also a difficult component of informed consent because it is often impossible to know in advance what the negative outcomes could be. But, just as you need to think about what a reasonable person (the standard often used in the law to determine whether what a professional did was acceptable or actionable) might consider a risk to protect yourself, you need to be direct and honest with your patients about reasonably foreseeable limitations and negative outcomes. Such negative outcomes should include both proximal ones (e.g., "It might be uncomfortable and distressing to talk about certain areas of your life") and distal outcomes (e.g., "As a result of our therapy, relationships you have with significant others may change," or "As a result of this assessment, you could be determined to be an unfit parent"—although the language you use to convey such an outcome need not be quite that stark).

5. Part of your discussion about the limitations of therapy or of an assessment process should include a statement that you can only draw conclusions and make recommendations on the basis of the information you are provided. You cannot be a mind reader, so it will be important that the patient be open

and candid with you. Without that, your service is very unlikely to be of much benefit. Of course, the patient has the option of declining to talk about a specific topic, if she or he is not ready to be open about it, but telling only partial truths or untruths is likely to be counterproductive.

6. An alert about any duty to warn that jurisdictional law may be required. Those usually involve either imminent and serious risk of harm to others or the presence of abuse of a child or vulnerable adult. We discussed this element in more detail in Chapter 7.

7. A statement about where any results, whether in the form of a formal report or in the form of therapy progress notes, might be sent and what the procedures are for sending information to others (more about this below). This should include a statement that once you have sent information to another individual, you cannot take it back and you cannot control what that individual might do with that information.

8. A statement that the patient or evaluee can choose to discontinue the service at any point without any negative consequences, other than a report that has already been approved by the patient will be sent with a description of what has been done and a statement, without judgment, that the individual chose not to continue/complete the process.

9. A statement that consultation with another professional, including an attorney, is acceptable before a decision is made whether to continue the service or not.

10. A statement that the client has a right to a nontechnical explanation of the services being provided and of any results or conclusions drawn (the latter would most often be appropriate in the case of a psychological assessment). In most instances (except some court- or agency-ordered assessments), the client also has a right to receive a copy of any report or clinical notes that are created.

11. A statement that the client has a right to ask any questions she or he has regarding the nature of the service and the potential consequences of receiving the service.

12. A description of the unit costs (typically, per hour fee) of the service, an estimate of the total costs of agreeing to receive the service, and a description of how billing is handled.

13. A statement of your policy and the law regarding maintaining confidentiality of information obtained.

14. A statement of how you handle a request that involves a change in roles. We discuss this point in greater detail in Chapter 7 (this volume) and below in the context of both the Lynn case and the John Smith case.

15. A statement of how you handle any conflicts or disputes that might arise during the course of the service.

16. A statement that the individual has a right to obtain a copy of the laws and rules governing the practice of psychology and to make a complaint to the licensing authority (with address and telephone number of the licensing board included) as required by law or rule.

17. A statement that the individual has a right to be free from any unlawful discrimination and has a right to expect that she or he will not be taken advantage of or treated in a way that is primarily for the benefit of the psychologist.

18. A clearly thought out policy regarding electronic communication, including Facebook, Twitter, or e-mail or other social media for communication, including use of fax or, even, telephone for sharing information. For example, how much time between sessions would you be willing to spend on the telephone with a patient? Are you reachable during evenings, weekends, and vacations? Those policy items should be clearly stated from the beginning of your professional relationship. You should be aware of and communicate any limitations to privacy in using any electronic means of communication.

Release of Information

Unless you encounter an exception discussed below, state laws and regulations, as well as the ethics of our profession, require you to seek your patient's consent to provide anyone information that you have acquired during an assessment or treatment session or sessions. As a result, it is essential to familiarize yourself with the basics of developing a clear form and the process used to obtain a patient's consent to release confidential personal health information when needed.

The privilege to keep the information private lies with the patient, and information can only be released with the permission of the patient, through either a signed release form or an action that brings the information into the public domain, such as filing a lawsuit, with the information obtained by the psychologist a basis for the suit. Obviously, in the case of an assessment requested by some outside party, whether an attorney, as in the case of Ms. Sanchez, or another professional, in the case of Mr. Smith, putting in the time to do the assessment and then not being given permission to send out a report would be problematic. What is one to do? One obtains permission upfront, with a statement that if the person chooses to withdraw from the assessment before it is completed, a report will be sent to the designated person based on the information that had been obtained.

As we discussed at greater length in Chapter 6, common exceptions to the requirement to obtain permission to release information are, namely, the following four circumstances:

a. To comply with mandated reporting laws in cases of serious and imminent threat to another person or abuse or neglect of a child or vulnerable adult,
b. when the release of information has been ordered by a court,
c. when the release of specific information is necessary to provide the psychological service, and
d. when records have been subpoenaed by a licensing board as part of an investigation of a complaint.

Figure B.3 in Appendix B contains an example of a generic release of information form that you are able to modify as needed.

For your self-protection, as well as clarity with your client, permission to release information should normally be obtained in writing. Getting permission to release information is fundamental to our practices because without it no one could be assured of being able to trust us and people would not, therefore, be willing to share with us their private thoughts and feelings.

Insurance coverage is a special case. Logically, one would think that if patients want to use their insurance to cover the cost of your services, they would expect you to comply with the coverage requirements of the insurance company. That may not always be the case, however. This is an example of a situation that can be, at best, awkward for you, even though you have not really done anything wrong. Thus, the best practice is to obtain from every patient who wants to use insurance coverage a signed limited release of information form to allow you to share the information required by the insurance company for them to pay you.

The following elements will provide you guidance in the development of a release of information form and process to discuss this release with your patient:

1. The date the form was signed and the name of the patient.
2. The name, address, and phone number of the person being granted permission to release information.
3. The name, address, and phone number of the person who is to receive the information.
4. A statement that the patient has a right to maintain privacy of all information and is under no obligation to sign the form.
5. The specific information being authorized to be released, the form of the release (i.e., copies of records, summary, verbal or

written information), dates of treatment or assessment, and limitations upon any disclosure.

6. The reasons the information is being released.
7. The inclusive dates the release covers or that it automatically expires after 12 months or a certain period of time specified by law or rule.
8. A statement that the authorized release can be revoked at any time, with the exception that such revocation of permission does not cover any information that has already been released.
9. Signature of the patient authorizing the release and, if not the patient, the authority the signatory has for signing.
10. A statement that information obtained is considered confidential and except with specific exceptions, information will not be released without the individual's expressed permission.
11. A statement of the potential consequences of releasing information. Although it is difficult to foresee all consequences, the following is a reasonable list. When you are in independent practice, it is a good idea to consult an attorney or other expert in your jurisdiction about releasing information if you have questions.
    a. Others, even beyond those designated in the release of information form, might obtain information that the patient would prefer they not know about him or her.
    b. The information release could have an adverse effect on any ongoing legal action.
    c. The information release could have an adverse effect on employment, job opportunities, or desired services or benefits.

Providing a well-designed informed consent process, using an easy-to-understand release of information form, and following HIPAA and state laws and regulations are excellent steps to manage risks that may occur in your practice. Certainly not all of the above events will occur, but the patient has a right to know with reasonable probability what could happen, so she or he can make an informed decision about whether to proceed with the release of information.

Now, let us turn our attention to the three cases we have been discussing. What are the specific risks involved?

Specific Risks

Although Murphy's Law (i.e., anything that can go wrong, will) does not really apply for any specific case, sooner or later in your career, some things will go wrong or minimally, will not go as planned. Risk management has to do with being able to anticipate what could go wrong and to respond effectively if it does. To explore possible risks in the cases we have discussed, it is helpful to ask yourself, What could possibly go wrong in the case of Lynn?

Case 1—Lynn

Clearly, the first and foremost thing that could go wrong in Case 1 is that as a result of the assessment and/or treatment of Lynn, her employability status is affected. That is certainly true if feedback is provided to the employer, an issue that is discussed in Chapter 7. However, it is also possible that her employability or employment status might be affected even if you do not provide any kind of feedback. That is, the employer who experiences stigma about psychotherapy could conceivably decide (maybe not rationally or fairly, but who says that rationality or fairness are considerations in a worst-case scenario?) that being treated by a psychologist is a tantamount admission that Lynn is not doing well. Because of a biased view about psychotherapy, the employer could decide to fire or suspend Lynn or to curtail her workload, any one of which could (and probably would) upset Lynn and, potentially, may lead her to blame you. So, what would be an appropriate risk management plan for such a scenario? There is no guarantee that any action on the part of a psychologist could influence the actions of the employer, so counting on his or her rationality and fairness is not a viable game plan. An appropriate risk management plan should rely first and foremost on actions you can take. Neither is deciding to send a positive report on the treatment back to the employer a viable option. First, even doing that is no guarantee that the employment outcome for Lynn is going to be positive. To trust in that is to rely on the actions of another person. Second, HIPAA confidentiality and privacy considerations are involved, as previously described. There is no ethical basis for sharing such information with the employer, unless the patient instructs you to do so, after you have had an extensive conversation with her about what the potential consequences might be of doing so, both positive and negative. Third, you should have the discussion about how to handle such a situation before the outcome is known. A patient might, potentially, decline to allow sharing of information and later change her mind, if the therapy process went well. That creates a different kind of dilemma for the psychologist, however. It puts the psychologist in the position of agreeing to release only positive information, which can create pressure to convey things in a positive light or, even, to be less than completely honest. One primary goal of risk management is to avoid situations that are awkward for the psychologist, or, even more importantly, place the psychologist in a situation which allows no good solutions, where either harm to the patient or to the psychologist are possible.

The only viable way of engaging in appropriate risk management in such a situation is to undertake a careful and complete informed consent process. We again emphasize that such a process is not primarily about providing a form to a patient and getting the patient to sign. Doing that may be consent, although, as discussed above, just having a patient sign a form in not adequate and truly informed consent. The informed part of the consent means that the patient understands what the options are and understands what the various consequences might be and, based on those understandings, makes a decision about how s/he wants to proceed. That does not reduce the risk to zero, but if you have engaged in such a process and carefully documented what you did, what the issues were, and what the decisions were and why, the probability that you will be held accountable for some negative outcome will be extremely low.

The second risk has to do with the possible outcome itself. The case history indicates that Lynn is concerned about the impact her psychological issues is having on her career and worries about losing her job. She is looking to therapy as a means of changing course and protecting her career. That is a considerable amount of pressure on you. Her life happiness and her vocational future depend on the outcome of the therapy. Again, informed consent is the appropriate way to manage that risk. Although there is research that indicates that a patient who has positive expectations of the therapy increases the likelihood of a positive therapeutic outcome (Constantino, Arnkoff, Glass, Ametrano, & Smith, 2011; R. P. Greenberg, Constantino, & Bruce, 2006; J. Miller, 2009), from a risk management perspective, these expectations have to come from the patient him/herself. The psychologist who has testimonials on his or her website in an attempt to influence the expectations of patients and potential patients is not only acting unethically (see APA, 2010; Ethical Standard 5.05), the psychologist may be creating undue influence by using testimonials that come from vulnerable patients or former patients (and, all patients are vulnerable by definition; who wants to be a test case in court for whether the patient was vulnerable to "undue influence" or not?). The psychologist is not engaging in effective risk management if the patient has been led to believe that a positive outcome is next to guaranteed. Therefore, both the wisest and the most ethical approach is to be very clear about what the limitations of therapy are and not to make promises that are impossible to keep.

The third primary risk in this case where services are offered by a student, namely, you, is that the services are provided by a person who is, by definition, not yet competent enough to practice independently. The risk is that if the outcome in the future were negative, Lynn or someone close to her could make the case that the services provided were incompetent.

Let us say, for example, that despite her protestations regarding suicidality, Lynn ends up committing suicide. The accusation could be made not only that the service provided was incompetent, but had the provider of the service been competent, she would have been able to recognize that Lynn was suicidal and would have taken action to prevent a successful suicide. Imagine the somewhat unlikely, but not impossible, scenario of those close to Lynn being aware of her suicidality, but you, the graduate student, took her at her word that she was not suicidal, and then she subsequently killed herself. Imagine the following interaction with a licensing board member or attorney (actually, the following questions as stated are much more likely to come from an attorney than from a psychologist member of a licensing board). How would you respond to these questions? Would you change the answers we provided in any way?

Attorney: Trainee A [i.e., you], you were not aware that Lynn was suicidal, is that true?

You: Yes, she told me she was not.

Attorney: And, Trainee A, were you also not aware that everyone who knows Lynn well did know that she was suicidal?

You: No, I was not aware of that.

Attorney: So, you accepted at face value her statement that she was not suicidal, is that correct?

You: Yes.

Attorney: You also diagnosed Lynn as having a major depressive disorder, did you not?

You: Yes. [Likely, using ICD–10–CM code F32.1]

Attorney: And, further, suicidality should always be considered in such a diagnosis, isn't that true?

You: Yes, that is true.

Attorney: And, further, despite the diagnosis, you accepted her statement about not being suicidal even though you state in your own records that Lynn was cautious about self-disclosing, is that correct?

You: Yes, but I also stated that she became more open and candid in her responses.

Attorney: Now, Trainee A, if she was cautious about self-disclosing at one point in the interview, isn't it possible that later, even though you thought she was more open, she reverted to being more cautious, especially if you were asking her about a behavior

	that could potentially result in your deciding you needed to hospitalize her against her will?
You:	No, I don't think she did that.
Attorney:	Trainee A, please just answer the question. I didn't ask you whether you thought she reverted to being more cautious, I asked you whether it was possible that she did.
You:	Yes, that is possible [because that is the only true answer you can give].
Attorney:	Do you have any specific tests or procedures that can tell you how open and candid or cautious a person is being?
You:	No [because there are no such tests].
Attorney:	Given that fact, did you ever consider contacting any of her family members and friends to make sure your conclusions about her suicidality were accurate? Isn't suicide a pretty important consideration where you would want to be very sure about your conclusions?
You:	Yes, it is important, but I didn't consider doing so, because I was taught that maintaining the patient's privacy was of primary importance.
Attorney:	So, you made the decision for Lynn that her privacy was more important than her life, is that what you are telling me? . . . I withdraw the question. [Thereby making the point without giving you an opportunity to respond.]

If you were given the opportunity to respond to this last question, what would you say? And how do you feel in this tough situation? No doubt you would be discussing your thoughts and feelings with your supervisor.

You get an idea of how such a process could go. This is a difficult dialogue with the attorney who has boxed you in. In your responses, the important and ethical way to respond is to be honest without extensive efforts to justify your oversight or error. Once you have missed something important, it is very difficult to go back and fix it. That is why a carefully considered and comprehensive informed consent process is important, both to increase the likelihood that Lynn will be candid with you and so that you can explain exactly what you communicated to Lynn about openness, as well as about the limitations of your efforts. It is also why using the ICD–10–CM as a means of determining what questions to ask and what possible symptoms/behaviors to pursue in your assessment process is so important.

Of course, another important element of your informed consent process should have been conveying the information clearly that you were a student in training, and that all sessions with Lynn would occur under supervision. Lynn would then have the opportunity to decline the professional service without negative consequences if she did not want to work with a student. That circumstance also has major implications for the nature of the supervision, that is, that you must be open and candid with your supervisor about all elements of your interactions with Lynn. All of us wish to hide those parts of what we do that we, upon further consideration, decide do not reflect well on us. In supervision this same phenomenon exists (Mehr, Ladany, & Caskie, 2010), which is exactly the wrong thing to do. It is precisely in those areas where you are weak that you need training, and it is by your commitment to professional development that you will communicate actions on your part that may be problematic that you maximize risk management. In supervision, if you only put your best foot forward, you may find that you step in potholes regularly. However, when you partner with your supervisor, she or he will be most effective and helpful to you to manage the risk of practice and to grow personally and professionally, particularly when you feel safe and supported and can discuss your professional concerns.

Case 2—John Smith

The first risk management issue in the case of Mr. John Smith is the same as the first ethical issue: Should you attempt to undertake an assessment with, potentially, limited access to data and with little idea of the specific goals of the assessment within a period of 2 weeks? The temptations to do so are great. You are in independent practice, and your livelihood depends on how much work you do (or, while in school, the quality of your training depends on the kinds of cases you see and supervision you receive). So, there is financial (or educational) self-interest in taking on this task. In addition, your relationship with Dr. Jones, and with the medical staff of this hospital more generally, could possibly depend on whether you accept this referral, and that also could have more long-term financial implications. It is very difficult to make wise choices when the consequences for you are as dramatic as they could be in this case. Clearly, the easiest thing to do from a risk management perspective is to decline the referral. However, risk management does not and cannot mean that you reduce the level of risk to zero.

So, what do you do in this case? The most important thing is to engage in an initial process of deciding whether you can, in a reasonably competent manner, conduct the assessment and answer the referral question you have, which is "to determine a psychological diagnosis and possible disposition." The case describes some methods for gathering the information necessary to answer your own question about whether you should accept the case. The best risk management strategy is to go through those methods and then be honest with yourself about what the reasonable thing to do is. Doing that creates another complicating factor, however. If you call Dr. Jones's office and read through the chart and then decide you cannot reasonably conduct a competent assessment, the time you spent gathering the necessary information might well not be reimbursable, that is, you will have just donated your time. Based on your own value system and on Principle B of the APA Code of Ethics (2010), you might well decide to provide some service pro bono, that is, without remuneration, but you likely will want to have more control over when you do that than this case allows.

This situation highlights one important general risk management component: If you are in independent practice, do not think first and foremost about the financial implications of clinical decisions you make. Doing so will almost certainly lead you into very dangerous waters sooner or later. You must believe that you will be able to earn a decent living by behaving in an ethical and competent manner, and that, in fact, long term you will be much better off, professionally and financially, if you do so. You do not need to be aware of every billable minute or, even, billable hour, for that billable time to accumulate to a level that at the end of the month or year, you have earned enough to make a living. So, when you confront dilemmas, think first about the ethical considerations, that is, what do the ethics codes say, what do the laws and rules in your jurisdiction say, and what is in the best interest of the patient. Second, think about how best to protect yourself from possible negative outcomes. In the vast majority of cases, if you focus on the ethical issues of practice, you will develop a positive reputation among providers and the financial aspects of practice will fall into place.

The second risk management issue involves your relationship with others at Mr. Smith's place of work. Do you have a conflict of interest because your sister's significant other works in the same company as Mr. Smith? Will your relationship with your sister's significant other or your sister, for that matter, influence how you will proceed with this case?

What is the worst possible outcome if you accept this case? One negative outcome could be that you write something in your report that reflects badly on Mr. Smith. It really wouldn't matter what it might be, but say you make a statement that Mr. Smith's ambition is interfering with his health (probably not a great statement to make in any case, because ambition itself is not a behavior that can be observed, so you are making an inference, and you can't know for sure that some internal state is causing Mr. Smith's medical problems). Mr. Smith is not furious about that statement, although he doesn't much like it. He subsequently finds out what the nature of your relationship is with your significant other's brother, Mark. He then makes the allegation that you were biased by that previous relationship and brings a complaint to the Board of Psychology. How would you defend yourself against such an accusation? It would be difficult. You could contend that you were not biased by your relationship with Mark, but it would be a hard thing to prove. If your assessment turns out to be pretty universally positive, the risk is likely to be very low. But, you can't know from the beginning whether your report will feel good to Mr. Smith or not, and the very last thing you want to do is to allow your concerns about how Mr. Smith might view your report to color what you write. That truly would be bias in your own self-interest.

Again, the safest strategy would be to decline the referral for reasons of a conflict of interest. However, depending on the setting in which you work (say, a relatively small community, whether a small city or small community within a large city), it could be difficult to avoid all such conflicts of interest. The issue is not to avoid all risk, but to take the best steps to manage it. Therefore, the second best risk management path for you to take (after being honest with yourself about not allowing your self-interest to determine your course of action) would be to consult with colleagues, just to make sure that you are thinking clearly and objectively about the situation. And, as we mentioned with regard to supervision when discussing the case of Lynn, consultation with colleagues is not likely to be of maximum benefit to you unless you are frank with them about the situation and your reactions to it.

The third risk management issue in this case is making sure that you are competent to provide the psychological service being requested. Although discussed previously at some length, it does bear repeating that one of the best risk management tools you have is only to practice within your areas of competence. Let us say that Mr. Smith is mildly unhappy with your report and then finds out about your relationship with Mark and accuses you of bias to the licensing board. If the report you wrote is done competently, with a basis for your conclusions in the data you have (remember the five potential sources of data we discussed in Chapter 3), then another psychologist, such as a member of the licensing board, will be able to look at the data, compare the data with your report, and conclude that your statements and conclusions are reasonable. So, clear documentation and close adherence to the data are two very important risk management tools.

Another element of providing a competent report in this case has to do with not trying to do too much, not trying to be too helpful. The referral question is quite vague. Therefore, you do not know exactly what Dr. Jones is looking for. The temptation is to try to provide as much information and as many conclusions as possible, hoping that the shotgun approach will at least hit part of the target. That is often a bad idea, because you stretch yourself to say things that may not be adequately supported by the data you have acquired. Beware of good intentions that are not based on good information and good judgment!

The issue of informed consent is also involved in this case. The most important aspect of risk management regarding informed consent is ensuring that the consent is truly *informed.* That means having a thorough discussion regarding the services and their risks and limitations involved (and potential benefits, but describing potential benefits is not a necessary risk management strategy), so that Mr. Smith can make a decision based on all of the information he needs to decide for himself how and if he wants to proceed. When seeking Mr. Smith's consent for the assessment, it would be beneficial to use the steps in the process outlined earlier in this chapter.

The issue of self-disclosure may also be an issue of potential risk. How much and what kind of self-disclosure is ethical and appropriate? This is a situation in which there is no easy answer and it is dependent on your theoretical orientation and previous supervisory experiences. And, there really are no clear standards to help us know exactly how much to disclose, in large part because it will depend on what Mr. Smith wants to know and how much self-disclosure would be beneficial to build a trusting professional relationship. It will also depend on how much self-disclosure is too much for Mr. Smith. At what point would he be inclined to say (even if his statement is unfair and a misrepresentation), "All the psychologist did was talk about himself [or herself]" (an unfortunate, but not infrequent, comment from patients). On the other hand, does Mr. Smith have a right to know about your relationship with Mark? Probably, yes.

It might well be that the best risk management approach is to determine how best to approach Mr. Smith regarding self-disclosure, keeping in mind what is in Mr. Smith's best interest (Bridges, 2001; Sue & Sue, 2003). Perhaps limiting self-disclosure when it might be helpful would create a different kind of risk, namely, a lack of trust in the professional relationship, resulting in a lowered motivation on Mr. Smith's part to be open and candid with you. The best strategy, in our opinion, is to be careful about what and how you self-disclose, always trying to focus on what is in the patient's best interest. Be willing to answer personal questions (which actually are posed by patients relatively infrequently) as directly as you can, being aware that revealing too much or too little about yourself has its own risks.

Case 3—Anne Sanchez

The case of Ms. Anne Sanchez presents multiple opportunities to manage risk. She has lived a difficult life and has made a number of choices as she seeks to survive in a very difficult world. You may have certain reactions to some of the choices she has made. For example, let us assume that you are troubled by her former lifestyle, because of your ethical principles or religious upbringing, or perhaps because you are genuinely concerned about what impact her lifestyle has had on her. And, perhaps you are a person who does not hide such feelings well, so Ms. Sanchez knows you are minimally uncomfortable or, even worse, distressed by the decisions she has made and the life she has lead. How would you, or how could you, defend yourself against an accusation that you treated her in a biased manner because of her history? In addition, as we discussed previously, there is the important ethical question of whether you have sufficient knowledge of Ms. Sanchez's history and how that might impact her psychologically. If you do not have this understanding of the issues she has faced in her life, you could be accused of practicing outside your area of competence. Unless you have gained competence, having the required knowledge, skills, previous experience, and attitudes that would enable you to assess and treat Ms. Sanchez, you may have difficulty as her psychologist.

The assessment that is being requested is very complex in that there are multiple problem areas for Ms. Sanchez. Are you competent in all of them? In our description of the case, we have you deciding that you are not sufficiently competent in neuropsychology and in chemical dependency to take on those two pieces, so you suggest a referral to someone with such competence. However, that still leaves depression, psychotic processes, and health psychology as specialty areas involved in this case. If you are not competent in those areas or cannot convincingly demonstrate such competence, usually through a combination of knowledge, experience, and supervision/consultation, it may be difficult for you to provide competent service to Ms. Sanchez.

Another potentially risky area has to do with payment for your services. Nothing is said in the case description about how or whether you will be paid for your services. If you had not thought about that when you read through the case, if you were in independent practice at some point you certainly would. And that point should be at the initial contact with the referral source and then when you have contact with the patient. If you discontinue a professional relationship when the patient needs psychological treatment or assessment only because you are not being paid, you could potentially be accused of abandonment for your own benefit. Ms. Sanchez is unemployed and was previously homeless, and is now living in her mother's converted garage. She is being assessed to determine whether she is eligible for financial aid, meaning she is probably not currently receiving any. She almost certainly is lacking in any substantial personal financial resources, and she may well be without any kind of health insurance coverage. If you decide to provide services to her pro bono, you should do that very intentionally and very consciously from the very beginning. So, you need to think through carefully what policies you will have regarding the provision of services to indigent individuals or individuals with significant financial problems.

Mind you, we are not recommending that you not do so. We also take seriously the APA (2010) Ethics Code Principle D, regarding justice, and the CPA Code (2000) Principle IV, regarding responsibility to society. We are simply recommending that you be clear, both in your own mind and in your communications with others, what your policies are, that is, how you will handle a whole host of situations involving payment for your very valuable services. For example, do you take on those who cannot pay at all? Do you continue to see individuals after their benefits or available funds are exhausted? Do you have a sliding scale, and if so, how do you determine what their income is, that is, do you trust whatever they tell you or do you require some kind of verification process? Do you require payment up front or will you bill them? Do you have a limit on the number of sessions/hours that they may be in the arrears before you take some kind of clinical or legal action? If yes, what would that action be? Do you use a collection agency, with whom you would have to share private information (name, address, amount owed, at a minimum)? If yes, have you informed your patient from the beginning about your policies? (You had better!)

Another major area of potential risk in this case concerns to whom you owe primary allegiance. The referral came from an attorney. Does that mean that the attorney is your primary client? Your only client? What do you do if the interests of the attorney and the interests of the examinee diverge? Let us say that the attorney decides she or he wants to keep some finding or conclusion of yours confidential, because it might be detrimental to the legal case. This is especially likely to occur if the assessment is a so-called adverse assessment, for instance, if you are hired by the state to show that Ms. Sanchez is not eligible for any kind of taxpayer support. But either you or Ms. Sanchez believes that it would be advantageous to her for that information to be made known. To whom do you owe allegiance in that situation? Would it matter, when such a difference in perspective occurs, who is paying the bill? We have written the case in such a way that Ms. Sanchez is unlikely to be able to pay for the assessment. However, if she were a person of means and was paying for it herself, would that change your allegiance? Or, if the attorney (e.g., the state) were paying you in an adverse situation, would that change your allegiance? This is a very complex issue that is dependent not only on state law but also on HIPAA regulations. Consultation with your own attorney to find out how best to proceed, if you have competing directions, is recommended. Our ethical perspective, however, is that both the referral source, especially if they pay for the cost of the assessment, and the examinee have a right to expect that you will act in an objective and reasonable manner, keeping in mind their best interests. The primary determining factor should not be who pays, but who the recipient of the psychological service you are offering is. In the case of Ms. Sanchez, it is both the attorney and Ms. Sanchez. As a result, you have a fiduciary responsibility to both.

Last, in this case with Ms. Sanchez, is one of the most emotionally charged of all issues: sexuality. Are you clear in your own mind how you will deal with provocative or flirtatious behavior such as that exhibited by Ms. Sanchez? The answer to that question needs to include not just, "I won't get sexually involved with a patient"; you will also need to know how exactly you will handle such a situation. Ms. Sanchez has acted in a flirtatious manner with you. How do you respond to her? How does that impact your assessment and your subsequent contacts with her, if any? How do you respond if she ups the ante and essentially propositions you? She is beginning to act in a provocative manner with you. Doing an assessment with her is likely to result in a different response than if you were providing her therapy. If her behavior is sexualized and she seems to be merely playful, does that influence your response? To what degree can you trust your own impressions regarding the seriousness and the intent of the behavior? This is a critical situation and one in which you must trust your feelings. What is the appropriate action to take that incorporates her clinical issues and your ethical obligations, thus minimizing the risk that you could be accused of sexually inappropriate behavior? If there is a risk, what can you do to gather data that will support your position that you did not act in a sexual manner? What kinds of records will you keep? If your records are too detailed, can you be accused of being titillated by your patient's behavior? How long should you keep your records? What is the general statute of limitations in your jurisdiction regarding a patient bringing a complaint or a malpractice lawsuit? Is the statute of limitations regarding sexual behavior different? If yes (and many jurisdictions do not have a statute of limitations for sexual contact between a professional and a patient/client), which records do you decide to keep indefinitely? Do you know or can you know who at some point in the future might accuse you of sexually inappropriate behavior? So, do you keep every record indefinitely, just those that note clearly sexualized behavior, or records of patients with whom you believe that there is some probability of such an accusation being made?

As you can see, there is an almost unlimited list of difficult questions that a risk-management-sensitive psychologist should ask himself or herself. It should be said that false accusation of sexual behavior are quite rare. Neither of us, in dealing with hundreds of complaints to boards of psychology, have ever seen an accusation of sexual behavior on the part of the psychologist when the evidence was anything other than very conclusive that such behavior did occur. So, it may be reassuring that such a false accusation is a low probability event. Assuming you practice in an ethical, competent manner, it is neither necessary nor helpful to be overly anxious about such an event. Nevertheless, thinking through the issues carefully will help you prepare to deal with as wide a range of challenging situations as is possible. One thing is sure: During the course of your career, challenging situations, of whatever nature, will present themselves from time to time. Your life will be considerably easier and your risk much lower if you know your clinical, legal, and ethical responsibilities and can think critically about what to do when the situation arises and then follow through and do it.

Disposition—The Assessment Is Done, What's Next?

9

This book is not primarily a book on psychological interventions, and yet, without some consideration of the issues that confront a psychologist who is developing a plan for disposition (i.e., dealing appropriately with an individual patient or a couple, family, group, or organization) that will result in an improvement in that individual's or group's circumstances, this book would be incomplete. At the same time, responding with psychotherapy, consultation, or referral to the needs of a patient is an issue whose scope goes far beyond the limits of this book. In this chapter, we provide an introduction to how to think about developing a plan for intervention.

You will be exposed to a number of treatment resources more fully in your other academic classes and during supervision as you work to develop intervention plans for your patients. As you begin supervised practice, it will benefit you and your patients if you have a working knowledge of these resources.

http://dx.doi.org/10.1037/14778-010
A Student's Guide to Assessment and Diagnosis Using the ICD–10–CM: Psychological and Behavioral Conditions, by J. Schaffer and E. Rodolfa

Evidence-Based Practice

We strongly support the movement in mental health that has come to be known as evidence-based practice. *Evidence-based practice in psychology* (EBPP) is defined by the American Psychological Association Presidential Task Force on Evidence-Based Practice (APAPTF; 2006) as follows: "The integration of the best available research with clinical expertise in the context of patient characteristics, culture, and preferences" (p. 3). EBPP takes into account *treatment efficacy*, "the systematic and scientific evaluation of whether a treatment works" (APAPTF, 2006, p. 5), and *clinical utility*, "the applicability, feasibility, and usefulness of the intervention in the local or specific setting where it is to be offered" (APAPTF, 2006, p. 5). This movement is certainly not without its critics, on the basis of both a philosophy of science perspective (see Uebel, 2011; Weinberg, 2001) and a more direct critique of its use in clinical practice (see Chambless & Ollendick, 2001; Pagoto et al., 2007; Stiles et al., 2006; Straus & McAlister, 2000; Weston & Morrison, 2001). We believe that although there are faults in our current scientific methodology, it provides the best objective data that we have and that practicing without taking evidence-based practice models into account constitutes a potential risk to the public, questionable ethical behavior, and in turn a regulatory risk to the practitioner.

What does it mean to practice using an evidence-based model? First, it means to conduct a competent assessment, based on the available literature on assessment (see Hunsley, 2007), that is, an evidence-based assessment, the primary focus of this book. As you now know, using the Clinical Modification of the *International Statistical Classification of Diseases and Related Health Problems* (ICD–10–CM; National Center for Health Statistics, 2015) is one important means of providing an internationally accepted foundation for thinking about the appropriate questions to ask and the appropriate means for collecting data.

Second, using an evidence-based model means consulting the treatment literature to guide your treatment planning. Elements of practice that are consistent across models include developing a positive working alliance with your patient and doing an ongoing assessment as the treatment is being applied. This suggests that if the treatment is not helping, the psychologist should revise the treatment plan to another evidence-based model if it is available. If another model is not available, consult with a colleague to determine the next step in the treatment or refer to another therapist who may work from a different therapeutic modality. Thus, ongoing treatment planning is based on the ongoing assessment of the patient, which is, in fact, the most important component of evidence that the psychologist has (Woody et al., 2004).

One can consult a large number of resources when attempting to practice on the basis of the available evidence. Multiple texts provide an overview of the literature on psychological practices that have empirical support. We describe a few of these in Chapter 10, on resources for the practicing psychologist. It is important to mention here that APA's Division 12 (Society of Clinical Psychology) created a task force to review the scientific literature regarding empirical support for psychological treatments. The task force defined three categories of treatments: well established, probably efficacious, and experimental (Society of Clinical Psychology, 1993). The specific criteria for inclusion in the well-established and probably efficacious categories are clearly defined but are too complex for inclusion here (see Society of Clinical Psychology, 1993, p. 10). This report has been criticized on a number of grounds, not the least of which is that the favored approach of a given critique writer was not included in the list of well-established treatments.

In addition, there was a sense that the task force did not take into adequate consideration what has been referred to as the *common factors in psychotherapy*, primarily those components of psychological treatments that have to do with the professional relationship (see Duncan, Miller, Wampold, & Hubble, 2009, and Norcross, 2011b). Partially in response to that critique, APA's Division 12 and Division 29 (Psychotherapy) formed a combined task force (Norcross, 2011a) to explore this critical issue. The conclusions of that task force include the following two crucial points: (a) The therapy relationship accounts for why patients improve (or fail to improve) at least as much as the particular treatment method, and (b) The therapy relationship acts in concert with treatment methods, patient characteristics, and practitioner qualities in determining effectiveness. Thus, a comprehensive understanding of effective (and ineffective) psychotherapy will consider all of these determinants and their optimal combinations.

In addition, the joint task force listed those elements of the professional relationship that fall into one of three categories: demonstrably effective, probably effective, and promising but insufficient research to judge. For example, the three Truax and Carkhuff (2007) variables mentioned in Chapter 8 fall in all three categories: Empathy is categorized as demonstrably effective, positive regard as probably effective, and congruence/genuineness as promising but insufficient research to judge. A general conclusion/recommendation of the task force is that "concurrent use of evidence-based therapy relationships and evidence-based treatments adapted to the patient is likely to generate the best outcomes" (Norcross, 2011a).

At the same time that we place considerable emphasis on evidence-based practice, it is important to point out that we have much to learn about psychological interventions from scientific study. Psychologists are at an early stage in understanding scientifically the process and elements of psychotherapy. That might be surprising, given that one of the first texts that reviewed the scientific literature in psychotherapy was published in 1971 (Bergin & Garfield, 1971) and used by both of the authors of this text in graduate school. However, because so many variables have an impact on therapy outcome, a great deal of work continues to be needed to explore comprehensively the effective components of psychotherapy. This is surely one area in which practice needs to inform science as much as science needs to inform practice. In addition to the work of these task forces, there are 17 guidelines promulgated by APA that provide psychologists an overview of relevant issues in the treatment of specific populations or the provision of psychological services. These guidelines are accessible from the APA website (http://www.apa.org/practice/guidelines/). Applicable to the specific cases discussed in the previous chapters in this text are the following six guidelines: (a) Guidelines on Multicultural Education, Training, Research, Practice, and Organizational Change for Psychologists, (b) Guidelines for Psychological Practice With Girls and Women, (c) Record Keeping Guidelines, (d) Specialty Guidelines for Forensic Psychology, (e) Guidelines for Psychological Practice in Health Care Delivery Systems, and (f) Guidelines for Prevention in Psychology. Please see Chapter 10 of this volume for a description of these guidelines and where to find them. In addition to these resources developed by the APA and its Divisions 12 and 29, the Canadian Psychological Association developed a helpful resource, "The Efficacy and Effectiveness of Psychological Treatments," also described in Chapter 10.

These documents provide a broad foundational overview of treatment issues, utility, and efficacy that the practicing psychologist can integrate into his or her practice. As Norcross and Wampold (2011) stated, psychotherapy is increasingly effective when the therapy is tailored to the individual as "different types of clients require different treatments and relationships" (p. 131). Thus, a psychologist will constantly make professional judgments about what the patient needs and how the psychologist will respond.

Treatment and Theory

In the process of learning how to be a psychotherapist, some students just want to be told what to say and how to say it during specific or difficult circumstances with patients. And to a new student entering an initial practicum training experience, almost all patient contacts are difficult circumstances.

However, psychotherapy does not work that way—and that is a good thing. Because every individual is different and presents with a different set of complex issues, a competent psychotherapist must be able to think critically and react to the unique presentation of each patient. Thus, diagnosis is an important element of the picture, both knowing what questions to ask, as we have described, and in the final formulation of who the person is. However, by itself, diagnosis is not sufficient. Hence, there are only labyrinthine paths involving a consideration of the complexity of the person in the development of a treatment plan. To develop a viable treatment plan, the competent psychologist must have a firm foundation in theory. That is required for two major reasons. First, as we discussed in Chapters 2 and 3 (this volume), a psychologist is able to obtain an enormous, and sometimes overwhelming, amount of information during the assessment process. Large amounts of data have little meaning or significance in the absence of a system for organizing and interpreting them. We argued in earlier chapters in this text that the ICD–10–CM provides an excellent starting point for doing so. Psychological theories provide a basis for understanding complex data and for providing a foundation for knowing the important questions to ask. Psychological theories also provide a basis for deciding what type of interventions should be pursued. Even the rather stringent criteria of the Division 12 Guidelines (Society of Clinical Psychology, 2014) do not point directly to specific behavioral interventions, given, for example, that for treatment of depression there are six approaches that are deemed to have strong research support and an additional seven approaches that have moderate research support. However, it is also not the case that all treatments are equal (the so-called Dodo bird hypothesis, based on Lewis Carroll's *Alice's Adventures in Wonderland*, in which the Dodo bird proposes a race where everyone runs whatever course they want, so "EVERYBODY has won, and all must have prizes," Carroll, 1865, p. 412). In fact, some have been shown to be harmful (Mohr, 1995; Ogles, Lambert, & Sawyer, 1995). Therefore, we believe that as you develop your theoretical orientation, it is important to incorporate the recommendations from the EBPP movement. It is critical to consider the empirical literature because a competent psychologist's theoretical orientation will influence the intervention plans for his or her patients. By way of full disclosure, the authors of this text have been most influenced by the theories describing behavior therapy, cognitive behavior therapy, and family therapy.

Standard of Care

An important concept in assessing and treating your patients is the standard of care. Many students and interns, as well as seasoned practitioners, even after a number of years of education, training, and practice, do not understand clearly what the standard of care is and how it is developed.

The *standard of care* is simply the level of care that a psychologist must provide after the development of a patient–psychologist relationship. The standard of care is a threshold of professional practice; it is not aspirational. It is the floor, not the ceiling. It is a legal term, developed as a result of various legal cases, that is generally defined as the practices that a reasonably prudent psychologist would adopt. The standard-of-care language originated in a British tort case (Bolam v Friern Hospital Management Committee, 1957, which has to do with the suffering that resulted from broken bones caused by electroconvulsive therapy for depression) and has set a standard that describes what the general professional community defines as appropriate practice.

Numerous influences help us as psychologists create the standard of care, including our theoretical orientation, the ethics codes of our professional association, rulings of the courts, regulations by state and federal governmental agencies, the current research literature, our training—in particular, our clinical supervisor's theoretical viewpoint—our patient's characteristics, our own biases, perceptions and characteristics, and the agency policies and procedures where we work. As can be seen, the development of the standard of care is complex and needs to be taken into account as we develop treatment plans for our patients. So, keeping in mind the scientific literature, theoretical perspectives, and standard of care, and the three very different patients we presented in Chapter 4 and discussed in the subsequent chapters, we are now able to explore what types of treatments and relationships might help them make progress toward their goals.

Case 1—Lynn

We conceptualize disposition in this case to involve psychotherapy, given the focus of the original referral. One result of the assessment that was done was that Lynn could benefit from psychological interventions. For the purposes of this exercise, we are going to assume that you (and we) have the competence required to provide the recommended psychological treatment. What follows, then, is an exploration of the issues to be considered and the thought process involved in organizing what hopefully would be a successful treatment plan for Lynn.

Let us start with a review of what we know about Lynn that may be relevant to disposition. This is best done in writing if you are new at creating an intervention plan. An excellent beginning point is to think about Lynn's differential diagnosis.

We discussed the implications of Lynn's signs and symptoms in Chapter 4. We mentioned a number of diagnostic possibilities for Lynn, some of which included Major depressive disorder, single episode of either a moderate (F32.1) or severe (F32.2) type, Generalized anxiety disorder (F41.1), and Adjustment disorder with mixed anxiety and depressed mood (F43.23). On the basis of the information that we currently have, we are not able to make a definitive diagnosis. A psychologist should only make a diagnosis when there is sufficient evidence for that diagnosis. Part of the message for disposition is that more work is to be done in gathering additional information, in line with the questions we asked in Chapter 4, before a complete intervention strategy can be developed. However, what are the specific signs and symptoms that lead to these differential diagnoses, and do they provide us with any ideas regarding disposition?

For this case, let us list Lynn's signs and symptoms in a visually succinct manner:

- recently changed behavior;
- growing sense of dread;
- decreased work productivity;
- lack of energy;
- difficult to leave home and go to work;
- decreased physical activity with mild shortness of breath;
- sad mood;
- displays visible signs of anxiety;
- communicates feelings of helplessness;
- use of alcohol, possibly as a self-tranquilizer; and
- difficulty with concentration and focus.

In addition to these specific signs and symptoms, what have we identified as important factors that are contributing to Lynn's referral for psychological services? Although we do not have definite answers to the following questions, they do shed some light on how we might think about formulating an intervention strategy. These questions explore both Lynn's strengths and areas of concern.

- How does Lynn understand the nature of her problems?
- Are Lynn's problems primarily related to work or do they extend into other areas of her life?
- What specific goals does Lynn have in seeking psychological care?
- Has she identified specific behaviors she would like to change?
- Does she have any thoughts about what would be helpful to her?
- How does she experience her growing sense of dread?
- What thoughts or experiences does she link to her feeling of dread?
- Where does Lynn turn for support or guidance?
- What or who are the potential sources of support in Lynn's life?
- What has been helpful to Lynn in the past when she has experienced similar feelings?

▪ How much social support, that is, supportive interpersonal rela-
tionships, does she have or does she allow herself to experience?
▪ How much disruption is there in her life from her symptoms?
▪ What does she do well and what is going well in her life?
▪ In which parts of her life does she feel in control and out of
control?
▪ What are Lynn's major vulnerabilities?
▪ What environmental triggers result in her emotional, behavioral,
and cognitive difficulties or dysfunctions?

As can be seen, we have many questions about Lynn's strengths
and weaknesses. In addition, we will want to better understand her life
and life circumstances at this point to help us search for an effective
intervention strategy. We know the following facts:

▪ Her mother, to whom she was close, died 2 months ago.
▪ An important relationship ended 5 months ago as a result of her
boyfriend becoming involved in a sexual relationship with someone else.
▪ She lives alone.
▪ She has a positive relationship with her sister, who, however,
lives some distance from her.

Obtaining answers to these types of questions will provide us with
the foundation to arrive at the best ICD–10–CM diagnosis and to begin
to develop an appropriate treatment plan. But, even distilled down,
the amount of information and the number of questions we have may
feel overwhelming. How does one begin to make sense of all of this
information? One excellent way is to think in terms of three categories
of human experience: affect, behavior, and cognitions. How can we
understand each of these, given the data we have, and where does that
lead us?

▪ *Affect.* We know that Lynn is unhappy and anxious about her
future. There are other indicators related to those emotions, such
as feelings of helplessness and a growing sense of dread.
▪ *Behavior.* We know her behavior has changed recently, although
we don't know much about exactly how; she has difficulty getting herself to work and she is less productive at work (also a
somewhat vague sign, so one that needs follow-up); she has had
a number of losses lately (mother, boyfriend, work productivity);
and she lives alone. We can hypothesize that some of these, such
as her losses, might trigger her current emotions, but we need to
find out more.
▪ *Cognitions.* We know perhaps the least about her cognitions, so
mostly, we have questions. We know she has had increasing dif-

ficulty with concentration and her sense of dread certainly has cognitive elements, although we do not know what those are. We think she might be resistant to therapy, although what that might involve, we do not know. We have much to learn about how she conceptualizes her life, her goals, her problems, her abilities, and her vulnerabilities.

Thus, even after our assessment with Lynn, we have many more questions than we have answers, but this list can still provide us with an outline of a framework of how we might think about proceeding. We know from the literature that the development of a trusting and safe professional relationship is important (Norcross, 2011b). And, given the number of questions we have, that is exactly where we should start. It will be through exploring all, or many, of the questions we have, some of which are listed above and others we listed in Chapter 4, that we not only can gather useful information from Lynn, but we will also communicate our intentions to her. We will develop a professional relationship that will focus on her and her needs and will be one of respect and caring, one of honesty and openness, and one in which she can feel safe enough to reveal her vulnerabilities and explore her possibilities. This may be a big step for Lynn, but it is one that we will take together.

Beyond our efforts to develop a strong working relationship, however, we know that there are emotions Lynn experiences that are undesirable and disruptive to her, so they need to change. How can that happen? We know that simple catharsis is not always enough (Tavris, 1989), but it can be helpful when working with uncomfortable emotions (L. S. Greenberg, 2002; Society of Clinical Psychology, 2014). Lynn is going to need to be given a chance to talk about and explore her various emotions. Initially, in addition to gathering additional information, exploring her emotions might well be the primary focus of therapy.

We also know that corrective experiences are helpful in changing undesirable emotions (Castonguay & Hill, 2012). Therefore, sooner or later, exploring with her behavioral changes she can make in her life and in her environment, so that she can have more rewarding and satisfying experiences, will be important. Exactly what those changes might be are not yet clear to us and will need to be part of the therapeutic process, but almost certainly they will need to deal with the nature of her interpersonal relationships; the nature of her intimate relationships; the support she feels or does not feel; and her relationship with her colleagues at work, about which we also know little, except that she has become less productive in her work responsibilities.

In the cognitive arena, a whole host of possibilities need to be explored. The fact that Lynn feels helpless and has a growing sense of dread almost certainly means that she conceptualizes her life as difficult and even threatening, and that she does not believe that she has the resources necessary to cope effectively. To the degree that this hypothesis is correct, she may need to be taught some useful skills to help her cope more effectively (note well: it is still a hypothesis despite our statement that it is almost certain—do not ever let your confidence in your theory or in yourself let you forget that you do not really know until you know, that is until you get the information you need directly from your patient).

Some of those skills may be behavioral in nature. For example, how to relate to others more effectively or how to manage stress more effectively. Some of those skills are very likely to be cognitive in nature. How to think about herself and her life not only more effectively, but more realistically. What Albert Ellis (1973) and Aaron Beck (1967) in particular taught us is that people are not always very good about developing beliefs about themselves and their lives that are positive and well-grounded in reality. So, Lynn may well need to learn how to think in a more realistic way about herself, her skills, her challenges, and her environment and see both the positives and the challenges, see her strengths and the problems. Thus, for example, we might have as one treatment goal the development of more self-confidence, related to her romantic relationships with men. Perhaps a second goal would be to enhance her ability to work more effectively, and a third goal would be to truly grieve the death of her mother. Although these goals would be helpful to her, they are not yet enough. Treatment goals need to be specific, behavioral, and measurable to be of maximum benefit.

Let us take the first goal, to enhance her romantic relationships with men, as an example. Lynn reports lack of trust in relationships with men, given her recent painful experiences with a breakup a few months ago. Yet, she appears to develop such relationships. Thus, a few specific objectives of this treatment goal might involve helping her identify and modify her emotions and cognitions about herself and about potential romantic partners (remember the authors' theoretical orientation includes cognitive behavior therapy, so that frame is used as a basis for this discussion). Specific interventions would include validating her emotional experience and helping her challenge her negative automatic thoughts, and in turn, her intermediate and core beliefs about herself and about men. Interventions would also include steps for behavioral activation, asking her to reduce any negative reactions to loneliness, perhaps by accepting invitations or asking someone to join her for lunch or dinner. What these behavioral steps might be would depend very much on what she has tried, what she wants, what opportunities she sees available, what she is willing to try, and so on. The development of a treatment plan is an interactive process between you and your patient. Developing treatment plans based on the other two goals mentioned would be similar. The plan and intervention strategies must be developed collaboratively with the patient.

As you can see, this is not yet a comprehensive treatment plan, but it is a beginning, based on the information and questions we have. We might not even have enough information to know how to adjust our preferred theoretical approach to the needs of this particular patient, so we do not yet know whether we should emphasize intervention on the affective, behavioral, or cognitive elements of Lynn's presentation. What we hope this discussion does, however, is to provide a schematic, based on the information we have and the scientific literature, that shines a light on the way forward.

One general framework for most all treatment plans we develop will include the following four elements:

- Set well-defined and clearly understood treatment goals tied to the particular signs and symptoms that compose the ICD–10–CM diagnosis. More specifically, although treatment goals can certainly include changes in affect and cognitions, they should also have behavioral implications, that is, specific and concrete behavioral changes should be included. This is true not only to satisfy insurance companies, which often require such specific goals, but also to make sure you are making practical progress as you work with your patients.
- Have a discussion with your patient or patients beforehand about your and their treatment goals. Such a discussion should precede the finalization of the treatment goals, both so the patient has a chance for significant input into what the goals will be and also as a means of getting the patient's buy-in to the stated goals.
- Decide beforehand with the patient how progress toward treatment goals will be measured and evaluated. Again, that evaluation should be concrete, specific, and objective and should include the means by which progress will be monitored.
- Review the treatment plan on a regular basis (every five sessions, or so, give or take a session or two, depending on the specific circumstances involved) and make modifications as needed. These modifications should occur when treatment goals change, resulting from changes in the life circumstances of the patient; when progress has been made (or deterioration occurred); or when the specific goals of the patient change.

Case 2—John Smith

As part of the preparation for this discussion, we (the authors of this text) made a list of signs and symptoms for John Smith, along with questions we have and life circumstances we have assessed, similar to that provided above for the case of Lynn. Because of space limitations, we decided to discuss the major issues in disposition for Mr. Smith rather than provide those lists here. We do, however, recommend that you make exactly that type of list as you begin to think about how to proceed with Mr. Smith or any patient you are working with. What we provide here is a list of those characteristics or factors that seem particularly and directly relevant to the issue of disposition for Mr. Smith.

First we must say that we do not yet know what a "disposition" for Mr. Smith exactly means. The referral was requested to provide information regarding "psychological diagnosis and possible disposition." That could mean the provision of psychotherapy following the assessment, but for reasons already discussed, that should not be assumed from the beginning. As the psychologist providing the assessment, it is your responsibility to provide a competent and thorough psychological assessment. Focusing the assessment on the assumption that you will provide treatment afterwards is a conflict of interest and an ethical dilemma.

As we acknowledged in the discussion in Chapter 5, due to the limited information we have, it will be helpful to gather additional information by administering psychological testing. We do have some information about Mr. Smith, however, that could help us formulate an outline of a possible approach to treatment to include in the report for Dr. Jones.

What do we currently know about Mr. Smith? We know that he is a fairly highly strung person. We know this from an observation of his behavior, from the high expectations and high stress he regularly experiences, and from the amount of time he spends at work. His tension, which may well reflect an underlying anxiety disorder, suggesting a working diagnosis of Generalized anxiety disorder (F41.1). This diagnosis with accompanying emotions, cognitions, and behaviors will certainly need to be a major consideration in his psychological treatment, in particular because of its potential contribution to, or relationship with, his angina. So, what are the specific circumstances related to his tension?

- high job-related stress involving both long work hours and high expectations,
- major feelings of anxiety related to concerns about his health,
- high expectations of himself learned in his family of origin,
- feelings of self-doubt involving inadequacy and inferiority,
- mild financial stress, and
- minor family conflict.

On the basis of these six issues, what general recommendations are we able to provide in the psychological report? The first two major concerns listed above have an external quality, as well as internal implications. That is, the reality that his job is demanding and stressful and his health are realistic concerns. Those factors exist independent of Mr. Smith's personal reactions to them. His particular history and view of the world are unique to him and shape the way he experiences emotions and cognitions. Some people would respond to such concerns in a different, psychologically and medically healthier, manner. As a result, part of the intervention needs to focus on helping Mr. Smith understand how to perceive and manage the stressors in his life differently and more effectively. This will certainly involve working on making changes in his environment, as well as learning how to adapt his behavior and his thinking regarding those things in his life over which he has control and those over which he has no control. Two classic works that we, the authors of this text, have found particularly helpful are Lazarus and Folkman (1984) and Meichenbaum (1985; see also more recent literature: Barlow, 2014; Lehrer, Woolfolk, Sime, & Barlow, 2008; Mate, 2011; McGrady & Moss, 2013; Rehm, 2010).

The second two concerns, high expectations and self-doubt, are internal and not connected in an obvious way to Mr. Smith's presenting medical problems. This does not mean that the concerns are less important than the first two issues, but it may mean that Mr. Smith might be somewhat more skeptical of discussing something so personal. That is certainly an issue that the psychologist would need to explore with Mr. Smith. However, an effective treatment plan for his psychological issues would almost certainly need to include a review of his cognitions about himself and his life and work to help him develop more realistic and reasonable thoughts about who he is and what he does. This is an area in which cognitive behavioral approaches have been shown to be particularly effective (Butler, Chapman, Forman, & Beck, 2006; Hofmann, Asnaani, Vonk, Sawyer, & Fang, 2012; Hofmann, & Smits, 2008). An exploration of his childhood experiences, where he learned to create high self-expectations developing into his core beliefs about the world, himself, and his relationship with others, will likely need to be part of Mr. Smith's treatment.

The last two issues, the stresses he experiences in his family and with his finances, are also realistic ones for which both behavioral and cognitive strategies might be helpful. That is, one useful approach is a problem-solving approach (D'Zurilla & Nezu, 1999), consistent with what we said above regarding learning to control the things we can. In the case of conflict over child responsibilities by two very busy parents, couples therapy could also be indicated to negotiate how those responsibilities can reasonably be shared (see Stuart, 1980). In addition, it might be helpful for Mr. Smith to consider his cognitions about his realistic stressors. Based on the information available, we don't know much about what those cognitions are, but one could easily hypothesize that there is a certain amount of overreactivity present, a cognitive reaction that Albert Ellis (1973) referred to as *catastrophizing*. Additional assessment would be necessary to specify what his cognitions are and how they may contribute to his disease.

Overall, are there any other interventions that could be useful to help Mr. Smith deal more effectively with his concerns and life problems? We do not know much about Mr. Smith's experience in the inpatient unit, but issues worthy of psychological consideration often arise, either in the way a patient feels treated or concerns that the staff has about the psychological status of a patient. Therefore, although there may not be specific interventions to undertake in this case, consultation with a hospital staff member—or the staff of some other agency that is involved with a given patient—is warranted and, even, necessary to support the improvement the patient is making. In essence, without intervening in the environment, it will be challenging for a patient to make necessary changes. The behavioral way of saying that is that without some control over the environmental contingencies, behavior change has a low probability of occurring or of being maintained over time. Therefore, a psychologist should always think more broadly than just one-on-one individual psychotherapy and decide whether other resources will be useful to incorporate into the treatment plan.

Case 3—Anne Sanchez

The first issue regarding Anne Sanchez's case is to decide what *disposition* means. The referral question was very clearly restricted to the issue of her employability and involved providing a psychological assessment with report. We argued strongly in Chapters 7 and 8 that it is advisable to restrict oneself to the referral question, particularly in a case that could end up in court, and not attempt to perform a variety of roles—for example, moving from being in the role of evaluator to that of a therapist, or even more problematic, being in the role of therapist and then attempting to conduct a formal evaluation. As a result, we strongly contend that the evaluator in this case should not take on the role of the therapist, but rather, if therapy is indicated, should refer Ms. Sanchez to an appropriate mental health provider for needed treatment. This means that, as a practicing psychologist, you do not practice in a vacuum. It is critical that you know the referral resources in your community because you will need to refer or collaborate on treatment with these colleagues.

Thus, "disposition" in this case means providing a written report that answers the referral questions as best a psychologist can and making a referral, if necessary and appropriate, to another provider for treatment. A strong case can be made that in a case like this, based on a referral from an attorney with a specific referral question regarding employability, that a recommendation for referral for treatment is inappropriate. This could be the case for two reasons. First, it is stepping beyond the specific referral question, which in a legal context is often fraught with risk. Second, it is taking an (unasked for) position that could cause complications in the legal case. Let us assume for a moment that the referring attorney in this case works for the insurance company that is involved. Depending upon the kind of insurance involved (e.g., health vs. disability), if you make a recommendation for treatment, you may in effect be saying that there is a mental health disorder and treatment is necessary. The implication could be that the insurance company should be liable for the cost of that treatment. Depending on circumstances, such a statement may well guarantee that this is the last referral you get from that insurance company, as your report made their lives more complicated. The major point is that you need to understand not only the specific referral questions but also something of the context of the referral to avoid potentially damaging pitfalls.

But, you might argue, what if Ms. Sanchez really does need treatment? The answer is that in this case, given a number of factors, including the referral question, the referral source, your role as evaluator, and who is actually your client (as discussed in Chapter 8, Ms. Sanchez, but also the referral source), the determination of the necessity for treatment may not be your role. Your role may be just to answer the referral question and in doing that, you can and should discuss the psychological issues involved in the case, as they are relevant to Ms. Sanchez's employability. But you also need to remember that being a competent psychologist means recognizing the limits of what you do in the various aspects of your practice.

What if the referral comes from Ms. Sanchez's attorney, who is trying to advocate for her in response to a decision by the insurance provider (in this case, an agency of the federal government)? If you are contracted by her attorney, who is her advocate, certainly it is acceptable and appropriate for you to provide as much information as possible to that attorney to assist in that advocacy? We would respond, probably so, but possibly not. If a question about treatment had been included in the referral, some response to that question would be appropriate. In the absence of such a question, we believe it is better not to provide unasked-for information, unless you also know the background of the question, have expertise in that area, and have had enough communication with the attorney to know what he or she wants.

So, you may ask, if the referral does ask for a treatment recommendation, is it appropriate to state that psychological treatment is necessary?

We would still encourage you to be cautious. If you state in your report that treatment is psychologically necessary, you may be, in effect, providing more information than was requested, and that information may not be helpful to your referral source and, in turn, to your client. However, even if the information would be helpful to the referral source, it is still not an appropriate role to extend your report beyond the referral question. This is a complex issue, and we caution you in writing reports to respond to and focus on the referral questions.

What would be appropriate, when a recommendation regarding treatment necessity is not requested, is to provide a description of the psychological problems that are present and how psychological treatments could be of benefit to Ms. Sanchez, without stating or implying that such treatment is necessary. Focusing on the benefits rather than the necessity of treatment might provide the referral source and Ms. Sanchez latitude in the next step they take without overstepping the boundaries of your appropriate role.

So, in terms of disposition with Ms. Sanchez, we are left with writing the report, along the lines suggested in Chapter 6 and recommending three referrals to the attorney, two of which were also mentioned in Chapter 6. These referrals are for a neuropsychological assessment and a chemical dependency assessment, because it was decided that the evaluator did not have sufficient competency in those two areas. In this case, it can reasonably be assumed that a focused employability assessment will also be conducted, but in a different, nonforensic context; thus, a referral to an employment expert for determination of what types of employment might be possible for this patient would also be indicated. In a nonforensic context, a referral to a psychiatrist for determination of whether pharmacotherapy for her depression and hallucinations might also be indicated but has some risks in a forensic context, for reasons discussed above.

As is true with our discussion of ethical issues in practice, disposition is a major topic in the training of psychologists. We anticipate that you will have multiple courses in how to provide effective psychological interventions, and we encourage you to avail yourself of the expertise your supervisors have.

Resources—To Prepare for the Work of a Psychologist

10

This chapter briefly describes some resources we hope will be useful to trainees in psychology. It offers a snapshot of the material a practicing psychologist should know is available and should consult when needed.

We have decided to focus on the following resources: (a) the *International Statistical Classification of Diseases and Related Health Problems* (ICD; see, e.g., World Health Organization [WHO], 2016) and diagnosis, (b) additional resources for diagnosis, (c) assessment, (d) clinical interviewing, (e) practice guidelines, (f) evidence-based practice, (g) ethics and risk management, and (h) resource for other resources.

ICD and Diagnosis

Although the *Blue Book* (WHO, 1993) provides useful guidance for diagnosis, it is not as thorough, comprehensive, or up-to-date as a textbook on psychopathology. The ICD system

http://dx.doi.org/10.1037/14778-011
A Student's Guide to Assessment and Diagnosis Using the ICD–10–CM: Psychological and Behavioral Conditions, by J. Schaffer and E. Rodolfa

assumes a degree of expertise in diagnosis that the professional brings to the process of assessment. For additional information about the ICD, we provide you with these four easily accessible resources:

- *ICD–10 Classification of Mental and Behavioural Disorders: Clinical Descriptions and Diagnostic Guidelines*. This document, commonly referred to as the *Blue Book*, provides a description of the main clinical features of all of the mental health diagnoses in the ICD–10. This is free and accessible at http://www.who.int/classifications/icd/en/bluebook.pdf.
- *ICD–10–CM*. This manual and related documents, produced by the U.S. government through the Centers for Medicare and Medicaid Services (CMS) (2015a) and National Center for Health Statistics, is based on the ICD–10 and approved by the WHO, for use in clinical settings. The ICD–10 is intended primarily to provide a system for gathering health related data and as a common diagnostic system for research, whereas the ICD–10–CM is intended to provide a system that will track the presenting problem of every visit by a patient to a health care professional. The 2015 update of the ICD–10–CM is free at http://www.cdc.gov/nchs/ICD/ICD10cm.htm#ICD2015
- The U.S. government has provided a website through the CMS that offers up-to-date information about the ICD–10 implementation and use: http://www.cms.gov/Medicare/Coding/ICD10/index.html?redirect=/ICD10
- *A Primer for ICD–10–CM Users*, Washington DC: American Psychological Association. Dr. Carol Goodheart has written an overview of the implementation of the ICD–10–CM to help psychologists and other mental health practitioners comply with the federal law.

Additional Resources for Diagnosis

For additional information about diagnosis, most readers of this book have taken or will take a course in psychopathology that used textbooks, which along with supervised clinical experience, will help them achieve competence in diagnosis. For students who wish to gain additional foundational knowledge in diagnosis, the following commonly used, excellent texts are noted.

Beauchaine, T., & Hinshaw, S. (Eds.). (2013). *Child and adolescent psychopathology* (2nd ed.). New York, NY: Wiley. This text provides a thorough discussion of childhood and adolescent disorders and examines genetic, neurobiological, and environmental factors within a developmental perspective.

Beidel, D., Frueh, C., & Hersen, M. (Eds.). (2014). *Adult psychopathology and diagnosis* (7th ed.). New York, NY: Wiley. This text provides a comprehensive introduction to existing views of psychopathology and its use and relevance in practice.

Assessment

Antony, M. M., & Barlow, D. H. (Eds.). (2011). *Handbook of assessment and treatment planning for psychological disorders* (2nd ed.). New York, NY: Guilford Press. This text provides an overview of the science-based assessment and treatment planning issues for all major psychological disorders, with an extensive list of appropriate psychological measures.

Groth-Marnat, G. (2009). *Handbook of psychological assessment* (5th ed.). New York, NY: Wiley. This book has long been considered the introductory, graduate-level text on psychological assessment, covering a broad range of basic topics, such as interviewing, the foundational issues involved in assessment, and an overview of some of the major psychological tests used in assessments.

Rust, J., & Golombok, S. (2009). *Modern psychometrics: The science of psychological assessment* (3rd ed.). Florence, KY: Routledge. This book is a useful overview of the science behind competent psychological assessment.

Sattler, J. M. (2014). *Foundations of behavioral, social, and clinical assessment of children* (6th ed.). La Mesa, CA: Author. Often referred to as the bible of child psychological assessment, this text provides a comprehensive overview of the issues involved in a thorough assessment of children.

Clinical Interviewing

Fontes, L. (2009). *Interviewing clients across cultures: A practitioner's guide.* New York, NY: Guilford Press. This book offers useful guidance to help practitioners conduct effective interviews with culturally and linguistically diverse clients and patients. Strategies to avoid common cross-cultural microaggressions and misunderstanding are explored.

McConaughy, S. (2013). *Clinical interviews for children and adolescents: Assessments to intervention* (2nd ed.). New York, NY: Guilford Press. This valuable book provides guidelines for interviewing children and adolescents, as well as their parents and teachers, to assess school, relational, emotional, and family issues, in addition to problem behaviors.

Sommers-Flanagan, J., & Sommers-Flanagan, R. (2013). *Clinical interviewing* (5th ed.). New York, NY: Wiley. This comprehensive text on interviewing provides a practical guide to a wide range of interviewing situations, from basic to more advanced situations.

Practice Guidelines

Practice guidelines, approved by the American Psychological Association (APA), are developed to provide psychologists with specific information to guide their professional behaviors and conduct. Guidelines are not standards, which provide a mandatory code of conduct that can be enforced by the profession or by a regulatory body. Guidelines are aspirational and provide a behavioral frame and set of goals that psychologists should strive to attain. They are developed to enhance the practice of psychologists and the development of the profession. It is important to emphasize that guidelines are not intended to take precedence over the professional judgment of psychologists; they are developed to assist the psychologist in using their professional judgment.

APA has approved 17 guidelines (APA, 2014) for the practice of various aspects of psychology. To be approved by APA, guidelines must go through a rigorous process of development and then be approved by APA's Council of Representatives, its governing body (APA, 2002a). The following six guidelines appear to be most relevant to the practice of psychology broadly covered in this book or are particularly relevant to training.

■ *Guidelines on Multicultural Education, Training, Research, Practice, and Organizational Change for Psychologists* (2002b). This document addresses the United States' "ethnic and racial minority groups as well as individuals, children, and families from biracial, multi-ethnic and multiracial backgrounds" (APA, 2003).

■ *Guidelines for Psychological Practice With Girls and Women* (APA, 2007a). This document articulates guidelines that will enhance gender- and culture-sensitive psychological practice with women and girls from all social classes, ethnic and racial groups, sexual orientations, and ability/disability statuses in the United States.

■ *Record Keeping Guidelines* (APA, 2007b). "These guidelines are intended to provide psychologists with a general framework for considering appropriate courses of action or practice in relation to record keeping."

▪ *Specialty Guidelines for Forensic Psychology* (APA, 2012b). *Forensic psychology* refers to the practice of psychology when applying the knowledge of psychology to the law in addressing legal, contractual, and administrative matters.

▪ *Guidelines for Psychological Practice in Health Care Delivery Systems* (APA, 2012a). These guidelines address psychologists' roles and responsibilities related to service provision and clinical care, including teaching and administrative duties within a diverse range of health care delivery systems.

▪ *Guidelines for Prevention in Psychology* (APA, 2013). As these guidelines themselves describe, they "offer guidance to psychologists on several levels, including supporting the value of prevention as important work of psychologists and providing recommendations that give greater visibility to prevention among psychologists regardless of specialty area or work setting (Snyder & Elliott, 2005)."

Evidence-Based Practice

Barlow, D. H. (Ed.). (2014). *Clinical handbook of psychological disorders: A step-by-step treatment manual* (5th ed.). New York, NY: Guilford Press. This is a comprehensive text on major psychiatric disorders, including diagnostic criteria, assessment issues, and evidence-based interventions for each disorder, with a strong dose of practical clinical wisdom.

Castonguay, L. G., & Oltmanns, T. F. (2013). *Psychotherapy: From science to clinical practice.* New York, NY: Guilford Press. This text integrates the science and practice regarding the more common forms of psychological disorders by presenting the science associated with disorders and drawing clinical implications from that science.

Duncan, B. L., Miller, S. D., Wampold, B. E., & Hubble, M. A. (Eds.). (2009). *The heart and soul of change: Delivering what works in therapy* (2nd ed.). Washington, DC: American Psychological Association. This text discusses the evidence-base of the common factors in psychotherapy, including relationship factors and is a must read for all psychotherapists.

Lambert, M. J. (Ed.). (2013). *Bergin and Garfield's handbook of psychotherapy and behavior change* (6th ed.). New York, NY: Wiley. The classic and standard text for what research has shown us about what works and does not work in psychotherapy across the broad range of issues in therapy, including research issues, therapeutic factors, theoretical approaches, and special settings.

Norcross, J. C. (Ed.). (2011b). *Psychotherapy relationships that work: Evidence-based responsiveness.* New York, NY: Oxford University Press. The standard book on what the research shows about how the professional relationship contributes to change in psychotherapy.

Website for the Society of Clinical Psychology, APA Division 12 (Society of Clinical Psychology; http://www.psychologicaltreatments.org). This website provides a great deal of information about evidence-based practice, including the criteria they used for categorizing treatments as having strong or moderate research support. The site provides a tab that lists evidence-based treatments alphabetically and a tab that lists treatments that have research support for each of the major psychological diagnoses.

Website for APA Practice Directorate (http://www.apa.org/practice/resources/evidence/index.aspx). This website provides the APA Policy Statement on Evidence-Based Practice, the APA Report that appeared in the 2006 *American Psychologist* on Evidence-Based Practice in Psychology, and the Report of the 2005 Presidential Task Force on Evidence-Based Practice. These three resources provide a foundation for competent and effective practice based on the science of the profession.

Website for APA's Public Interest Directorate (http://www.apa.org/pi/families/resources/task-force/evidence-based.aspx). This website provides the report of the Task Force on Evidence-Based Practice With Children and Adolescents, which describes challenges in developing and enhancing evidence-based practice for families and children/adolescents.

Canadian Psychological Association's "The Efficacy and Effectiveness of Psychological Treatments," provides a wealth of information for the practicing psychologist. This excellent document is available online at http://www.cpa.ca/docs/File/Practice/TheEfficacyAndEffectiveness OfPsychologicalTreatments_web.pdf.

Ethics and Risk Management

ETHICS

Bersoff, D. N. (2008). *Ethical conflicts in psychology* (4th ed.). Washington, DC: American Psychological Association. This comprehensive resource presents ethical dilemmas encountered by psychologists as they assess, intervene, and conduct research. Dr. Bersoff provides helpful perspectives on critical ethical issues that have no easy answers.

Fisher, C. B. (2012). *Decoding the ethics code: A practical guide for psychologists* (3rd ed.). Washington, DC: American Psychological Association. Dr. Fisher, chair of the task force that revised the *Ethical Principles of Psychologists and Code of Conduct*, has written a book for students and psychologists to help them understand this code. This book provides guidance on professional behavior, how to avoid ethical violations, and how to protect the welfare of clients and patients.

Knapp, S. J., Gottlieb, M. C., Handelsman, M. M., & VandeCreek, L. D. (2012). *APA handbook of ethics in psychology.* Washington, DC: American Psychological Association. This two-volume set provides coverage of the philosophical foundations of professional ethics and a resource for ethical issues that can arise in virtually any context, including professional practice, education, and research.

Pope, K., & Vasquez, M. (2011). *Ethics in psychotherapy and counseling: A practical guide* (4th ed.). San Francisco, CA: Jossey-Bass. Psychologists will encounter many ethical dilemmas without obvious or simple solutions. This is a terrific book that not only explores the ethical issues we encounter as psychologists but also encourages us to explore our own values and attitudes, that is, who we are as psychologists.

Pope, K., Sonne, J., & Greene, B. (2006). *What therapists don't talk about and why: Understanding the taboos that hurt us and our clients* (2nd ed.). Washington, DC: American Psychological Association. Pope and his coauthors wrote this book to help psychologists explore the myths and taboos that interfere with their practice. The authors provide provocative questions to help practitioners assess who they are, recognize myths they hold, and challenge taboos that interfere with their ability to be authentic with their clients and patients.

RISK MANAGEMENT

Knapp, S., Younggren, J. N., VandeCreek, L., Harris, E., & Martin, J. N. (2013). *Assessing and managing risk in psychological practice: An individualized approach* (2nd ed.), Washington DC: American Psychological Association Insurance Trust. Some areas of psychological practice result in ambiguity regarding ethical practice and professional liability for psychologists. This book, developed by the American Psychological Association Insurance Trust, helps psychologists identify and understand ethical and legal implications of the practice of psychology.

Resource for Other Resources

We close this chapter by mentioning *PsycEssentials: A Pocket Resource for Mental Health Practitioners* (2012), written by Dr. Janet Sonne and published by APA. This useful book provides resource information on a range of practice issues having to do with assessment, intervention, ethics, and risk management. *PsycEssentials* also has a mobile app that has up-to-date information for a psychologist's practice.

Appendix A: Interview Protocol

Name:
Age:
Ethnicity:

REASON FOR REFERRAL

Symptoms: When first occur, what happening then; how cope with, effectiveness of coping; situational precipitants; thoughts, physical sensations, affect accompanying; effect on work, relationships, recreation; severity, when worst, best, situational or coping factors associated with; changes over time; effect on of talking about

FAMILY OF ORIGIN AND BACKGROUND

Where born and raised; Developmental history
Father, mother, siblings; relationships with family in the past; current relationships; early memories
Communication style/expression of affect; conflict resolution/ decision-making style
Rules/punishment; history of abuse; losses/traumatic experiences
Psychiatric history in family

INTERPERSONAL RELATIONSHIPS

Childhood relationships; Current friendships/supports
Relationships with opposite sex, sexual history
Present family situation—married, children, etc.
Nature of relationships
Child care issues—if work, or if return to work
Other significant relationships
Current living situation

EDUCATIONAL BACKGROUND

Schools attended, graduation dates
Academic performance
Behavior/learning problems; subjects enjoyed
Extracurricular activities; vivid memories
Role models; favorite, least favorite teachers

VOCATIONAL HISTORY

Work history, jobs, when
Reasons for changes in past
Ever fired?
Current job, relationships, satisfaction
Stresses—burnout, conflicts, dissatisfactions, expectations about future
Quality of work performance
Quality of professional relationships
Vocational goals
Recent job seeking

INTERESTS/HOBBIES

Areas of enjoyment, recreation
Volunteer activities, past, present

SUBJECTIVE STRENGTHS/WEAKNESSES

Best thing done in life; worst thing done in life
What change in life if could
If three wishes granted, what would they be?

OTHER IMPORTANT LIFE EVENTS/ TRAUMATIC EXPERIENCES

CURRENT PSYCHOLOGICAL STATE

Mood, affect (duration, frequency, intensity)
Sleeping patterns

Appetite/weight changes
Concentration
Persistence
Memory
Sexual functioning
Energy level
Self-esteem
Suicidal ideation, strange feelings, feelings of hopelessness

LEGAL HISTORY

Juvenile record
Arrests, charges, convictions, sentences, parole

AGGRESSIVE HISTORY

Fights; how deal with anger

MEDICAL HISTORY

Major illnesses, high fevers, convulsions, poisonings
Injuries (head), unconscious, amnesia
Surgeries, anesthesia
Hospitalizations (birthing)
Developmental history
Pain/secondary gains, limitations on activity
Stresses related to symptoms
When first experience current symptoms/course
When seek treatment and why
Treatments and providers (addresses and phone numbers), efficacy
Treatment plan
Medications, past and present, dosages, response
On medical leave, job impairment, any improvement, anticipated
    return to work

PSYCHOLOGICAL TREATMENT HISTORY

Outpatient, inpatient dates, providers in past
When first experience current symptoms/course
When seek treatment and why
Treatments and providers (addresses and phone numbers), efficacy
Treatment plan
Medications, past and present, dosages, response
On psychological leave, job impairment, any improvement, anticipated
    return to work

CHEMICAL USE

Time of use, age, amount, frequency, physical symptoms, loss of control, treatment (inpatient, outpatient), current status

Alcohol, marijuana, hallucinogens, barbiturates, amphetamines, narcotics, cocaine, prescription medications

DAILY ACTIVITIES

Typical day (TV, music, reading, games, telephone, social events, movies, religious services)

Level of independence

Impairments

CURRENT FUNCTIONING

Personal hygiene (bathing, change clothes)

Cooking (frequency, types food, difficulties)

Cleaning (make bed, wash dishes, laundry, vacuum, mow lawn)

Shopping (frequency, make list, handle money)

Budgeting (handle own money, problems, jobs)

Mobility (drive, take bus independently, follow directions, get lost)

PERSONAL GOALS

Appendix B: Relevant Forms

Department

Agency

NOTICE OF PRIVACY PRACTICES

THIS DOCUMENT APPLIES TO HOW INFORMATION AND RECORDS REGARDING YOUR HEALTH CARE AT THE AGENCY MAY BE USED AND DISCLOSED AND HOW YOU CAN GET ACCESS TO THIS INFORMATION. PLEASE REVIEW THIS DOCUMENT CAREFULLY.

About us

The Agency is a teaching and research health care facility. All care is provided by a team of health care professionals. Residents, fellows, interns, students, and graduate students of health care professions schools may provide treatment to you or participate in examinations or procedures under the supervision of a licensed health care professional.

Example of the Privacy Practices Statement

FIGURE B.1 (*Continued*)

Your health care information

The Agency is committed to protecting counseling/psychological information about you ("health care information"). To the degree possible under the law, we will maintain confidentiality on all information you provide to us. We will generally only disclose your information when permitted by law or when specifically authorized by you. However, there are certain situations in which we are allowed or required to disclose information about you that you should know about. To the degree possible, even in these circumstances we will discuss disclosure with you before it happens. Please discuss your thoughts about these circumstances with your provider.

How we are allowed or required to use and disclose health care information about you

The following sections describe different ways that we are allowed or required by law to use and disclose your health care information. Some information, such as certain drug and alcohol information, HIV information, and mental health information, is entitled to special restrictions related to its use and disclosure.

- **For treatment.** When other agency personnel are involved in your treatment, such as supervisors or other health providers who are also providing services to you, they may have access to your health care information.

- **For payment.** We may use and disclose your health care information, including proposed treatment plans, to any insurance company or a third party you choose to use to cover the costs of the services provided you by the Agency.

- **Research.** The Agency is a research institution. All research projects conducted by the Agency staff must be approved through a special review process to protect patient safety, welfare and confidentiality. We may use and disclose information about our patients for research purposes, subject to the confidentiality provisions of federal and state law. That means, however, that your identity will not be revealed without your permission.

- **As permitted by law.** We may use and disclose health care information about you when required or permitted to do so by federal or state law, such as the following:

- **To avert a serious threat to health or safety.** We may use and disclose health care information about you when necessary to prevent or lessen a serious and imminent threat

Example of the Privacy Practices Statement

FIGURE B.1 *(Continued)*

to your health and safety or the health and safety of the public or another person. Any disclosure would be to someone able to help stop or reduce the threat.

- **Military and veterans.** If you are or were a member of the armed forces, we may release health care information about you to military command authorities as authorized or required by law.

- **Workers' compensation.** We may use or disclose health care information about you for workers' compensation or similar programs as authorized or required by law. These programs provide benefits for work-related injuries or illness.

- **Public-health disclosures.** We may use and disclose health care information about you for public-health purposes. These purposes generally include the following:

  - preventing or controlling disease, injury, or disability;

  - reporting vital events, such as births and deaths;

  - reporting adverse events related to food, medications, or defects or problems with products;

  - notifying a person who may have been exposed to a disease or may be at risk of contracting or spreading a disease or condition; and

  - notifying the appropriate government authority if we believe a patient has been the victim of abuse, neglect, or domestic violence.

- **Legal proceedings.** We may use and disclose health care information about you to courts, attorneys, and court employees in the course of conservatorship and certain other judicial or administrative proceedings.

- **Lawsuits and other legal actions.** We may use and disclose health care information about you in response to a court or administrative order, or in response to a subpoena, discovery request, warrant, summons or other lawful process.

Your rights regarding health care information about you

Your information is the property of the Agency. You have the following rights, however, regarding information we maintain about you.

Example of the Privacy Practices Statement

FIGURE B.1 (*Continued*)

- **Right to inspect and copy.** With certain exceptions, you have the right to inspect and/or receive a copy of your electronic health record (EHR).
  - To inspect and/or to receive a copy of your EHR, you must submit your request in writing to Custodian of Records at the Agency. If you request a copy of the information, there is a fee for these services.
- **Right to request an amendment or addendum.** If you feel that information we have about you is incorrect or incomplete, you may ask us to amend the information or add an addendum (addition to the record). Your request must be made in writing and submitted to Custodian of Records at the Agency.
- **Right to request restrictions.** You have the right to request a restriction or limitation on the health care information we use or disclose about you for treatment, payment, or healthcare operations. To request a restriction, you must make your request in writing to Custodian of Records at the Agency.
- **Right to request confidential communications.** You have the right to request that we communicate with you about health care related matters in a certain way or at a certain location. For example, you may ask that we contact you only at home or only by mail. To request confidential communications, you must make your request in writing to Custodian of Records at the Agency.
- **Right to receive an accounting.** Patients have a right to receive a record of specific types of disclosures made by the Agency. To request an accounting of disclosure, you must make your request in writing to Custodian of Records at the Agency.
- **Right to receive a paper copy of this document.** You have the right to obtain a paper copy of this document upon your request.

Complaints. If you believe that your privacy rights have been violated or if you have questions about your rights, you should contact the Agency Clinical Director. We will not take action against you for filing a complaint. Certain patients may also file a complaint with the Director, Office for Civil Rights of the U.S. Department of Health and Human Services.

Effective date July 1, 2015

Example of the Privacy Practices Statement

FIGURE B.2

Department

Agency

CLINIC INFORMATION AND TREATMENT AUTHORIZATION

Name:_____ DOB:_____

(please print legibly)

Welcome to our department. Our goal is to promote your health, growth, and well-being. Please review and sign this document, as it provides you information about important issues related to the services we provide. When you meet with your service provider, please discuss any questions or concerns you may have.

SERVICES AND ELIGIBILITY: Our department provides confidential, short-term psychological and psychiatric services to eligible individuals. The department does not provide assessment or treatment for legal purposes. Based on our resources, your individual therapeutic goals and your counseling needs, you may be referred to individual psychotherapy, group counseling, or to community providers for ongoing longer-term treatment.

STAFFING: Professional services are provided by licensed psychologists, psychiatrists, marriage and family therapists, and social workers. This facility trains psychology interns, residents and other health care professional trainees, who may provide services and participate in your care under supervision of a licensed health care provider.

CONFIDENTIALITY AND PRIVACY: Our staff will keep a summary of our contacts with you in an electronic mental health record that is maintained in a safe, confidential manner. Your information will only be released as permitted by law (for example, if you present an imminent danger to yourself or others; if there is a reasonable suspicion of child/elder abuse; if you are gravely disabled; if records are subpoenaed) or if authorized by you. The Agency Privacy Policy, which you received to review, identifies how your information may be used or disclosed.

APPOINTMENTS: Since demand for services is high, we ask that you only schedule appointments that you are confident you will keep. If you are unable to keep an appointment, please call our appointment line at least 24 hours in advance, so that we may make the time slot available to another individual seeking service. Please assist us in achieving maximum utilization

Example of an Informed Consent Form

FIGURE B.2 (*Continued*)

of this important health resource. Repeated rescheduling and/or canceling of appointments without advance notice will likely result in termination of care from this clinic. If staff cannot keep an appointment with you, or has other need to contact you, our staff will attempt to contact you by calling or texting the telephone number you provided and indicated that you preferred.

PSYCHOLOGICAL AND MEDICAL SERVICES WORKING TOGETHER WITH YOU:

The mission of the Agency is to enhance the physical and mental health of citizens in order to help them achieve personal development and lifelong wellness. To do this, psychology and medical providers work together in a team approach to promote your well-being, which may include the exchange of information. Medical providers follow a "need to know" guideline, which means that they will only access information in your psychological record if they believe it will benefit the care they are providing you.

TREATMENT AUTHORIZATION: I understand that the department provides psychology and medical providers who work collaboratively to provide health and mental health services. I understand that my mental health provider will collaborate with medical providers involved in my care, which may include consulting and sharing my treatment record, including psychotherapy notes.

_____ (initial) I have read this information about the department and give my consent to be treated by a health service student or licensed professional.

_____ (initial) I give my consent for my mental health information to be shared for the purposes described above.

_____ (initial) I was able to discuss any questions and concerns them with my provider prior to signing this form.

_____   _____

Signature   **Date**

You may request a copy of this form or the Privacy Policy at registration

Please return this signed form to the Registration Staff

Example of an Informed Consent Form

FIGURE B.3

Department

Agency

AUTHORIZATION FOR RELEASE OF PSYCHOLOGY CLINIC INFORMATION

Name_____Perm/ID #_____Date of Birth _/_/_

Phone_____Address_____

City_____State_____Zip code_____

I authorize:

(Person or facility which has medical and mental health information)

Name:_____

Address:_____

_____

Phone:_____

FAX:_____

to release medical and/or mental health information to:

(Person or facility to receive health information)

Name:_____

Address:_____

_____

Phone:_____

FAX:_____

Generic Release of Information Form

FIGURE B.3 (*Continued*)

Type of disclosure: ☐Verbal Information☐Copies of records☐Letter/Summary

Please specify the information you authorize to be released:

☐ Mental health information

☐ Medical (This may include drug/alcohol and mental health information documented by a primary care practitioner in the medical record)

☐ Drug and alcohol abuse, diagnosis or treatment information subject to federal law (42 C.F.R. §§2.34 and 2.35).

☐ HIV/AIDS test results (Health and Safety Code §120980(g)).

Type(s) of information, if not specified above (e.g. Summary Report)

_____

Specify date(s) of treatment, time period or condition:

Limitations upon disclosure:

The purpose of this release is:

☐ At the request of the client/patient/patient representative

☐ Other (state reason)

EXPIRATION OF AUTHORIZATION: Unless otherwise revoked, this Authorization expires

on: _____

If no date is indicated, the Authorization will expire 12 months after the date of my signing this

form.

Patient/Patient Representative Printed Name: _____

Client/Patient/Patient Representative Signature: _____

Date: _____

Relationship to Client/Patient: _____

Generic Release of Information Form

FIGURE B.3 (*Continued*)

NOTICE: This Agency and many other organizations and individuals such as physicians, psychologists, hospitals and health plans are required by law to keep your personal health information confidential. If you have authorized the disclosure of your health information to someone who is not legally required to keep it confidential, it may no longer be protected by state or federal confidentiality laws.

YOUR RIGHTS: This Authorization to release health information is voluntary. Treatment, payment, enrollment or eligibility for benefits may not be conditioned on signing this Authorization except in the following cases: (1) to conduct research-related treatment, (2) to obtain information in connection with eligibility or enrollment in a health plan, (3) to determine an entity's obligation to pay a claim, or (4) solely to create health information to provide to a third party.

This Authorization may be revoked at any time. The revocation must be in writing, signed by you or your client/patient representative, and delivered to our Agency. The revocation will take effect when the Agency receives it, except to the extent the Agency or others have already relied on it. You are entitled to receive a copy of this Authorization.

You have the right to receive written acknowledgment from a non-medical recipient of the information being released pursuant to this authorization agreeing to abide by the restrictions contained in this release. By signing here, you waive the right to receive such a signed written agreement from the intended recipient:

Signature_____ Date_____

Generic Release of Information Form

References

Abelson, R. P., Aronson, E., McGuire, W. J., Newcomb, T. M., Rosenberg, M. J., & Tannenbaum, P. H. (1968). *Theories of cognitive consistency: A sourcebook.* Chicago, IL: Rand McNally.

Ægisdóttir, S., White, M. J., Spengler, P. M., Maugherman, A. S., Anderson, L. A., Cook, R. S., . . . Rush, J. D. (2006). The meta-analysis of clinical judgment project: Fifty-six years of accumulated research on clinical versus statistical prediction. *The Counseling Psychologist, 34,* 341–382. http://dx.doi.org/10.1177/0011000005285875

Aetna. (2015). *Behavioral health provider manual.* Retrieved from http://www.aetnabehavioralhealth.com/i/A/ABHProvider Manual.pdf

Alarcón, R. D. (2009). Culture, cultural factors, and psychiatric diagnosis: Review and projections. *World Psychiatry: Official Journal of the World Psychiatric Association, 8,* 131–139.

American Psychiatric Association. (1952). *Diagnostic and statistical manual of mental disorders* (1st ed.). Washington, DC: Author.

American Psychiatric Association. (1968). *Diagnostic and statistical manual of mental disorders* (2nd ed.). Washington, DC: Author.

American Psychiatric Association. (1980). *Diagnostic and statistical manual of mental disorders* (3rd ed.). Washington, DC: Author.

American Psychiatric Association. (1994). *Diagnostic and statistical manual of mental disorders* (4th ed.). Washington, DC: Author.

American Psychiatric Association. (2000). *Diagnostic and statistical manual of mental disorders* (4th ed., text rev.). Washington, DC: Author.

American Psychiatric Association. (2013). *Diagnostic and statistical manual of mental disorders* (5th ed.). Washington, DC: Author.

American Psychological Association. (1990). *Guidelines for providers of psychological services to ethnic, linguistic, and culturally diverse populations*. Retrieved from http://www.apa.org/pi/oema/resources/policy/provider-guidelines.aspx

American Psychological Association. (2002a). Criteria for practice guideline development and evaluation. *American Psychologist, 57,* 1048–1051. http://dx.doi.org/10.1037/0003-066X.57.12.1048

American Psychological Association. (2002b). *Guidelines on multicultural education, training, research, practice, and organizational change for psychologists*. Retrieved from http://www.apa.org/pi/oema/resources/policy/multicultural-guidelines.aspx

American Psychological Association. (2003). Guidelines on multicultural education, training, research, practice, and organizational change for psychologists. *American Psychologist, 58,* 377–402.

American Psychological Association. (2007a). Guidelines for psychological practice with girls and women. *American Psychologist, 62,* 949–979. http://dx.doi.org/10.1037/0003-066X.62.9.949

American Psychological Association. (2007b). Record keeping guidelines. *American Psychologist, 62,* 993–1004. http://dx.doi.org/10.1037/0003-066X.62.9.993

American Psychological Association. (2010). *Ethical principles of psychologists and code of conduct (2002, Amended June 1, 2010)*. Retrieved from http://www.apa.org/ethics/code/index.aspx

American Psychological Association. (2012a). Guidelines for psychological practice in health care delivery systems. *American Psychologist, 68,* 1–6. http://dx.doi.org/10.1037/a0029890.

American Psychological Association. (2012b). Specialty guidelines for forensic psychology. *American Psychologist, 68,* 7–19. http://dx.doi.org/10.1037/a0029889.

American Psychological Association. (2013). Guidelines for prevention in psychology. *American Psychologist, 69,* 285–296. http://dx.doi.org/10.1037/a0034569.

American Psychological Association. (2014). *APA guidelines for practitioners*. Retrieved from http://www.apa.org/practice/guidelines/

American Psychological Association Practice Organization. (n.d.). *The HIPAA security rule primer*. Washington, DC: American Psychological Association.

American Psychological Association Presidential Task Force on Evidence-Based Practice. (2006). Evidence-based practice in psychology. *Ameri-*

can Psychologist, 61, 271–285. http://dx.doi.org/10.1037/0003-066X. 61.4.271

Americans With Disabilities Act. (2014). Retrieved from http://www.eeoc. gov/laws/types/disability.cfm

Anthem Blue Cross. (2013). *Behavioral health medical necessity criteria.* Retrieved from https://www.anthem.com/ca/provider/f1/s0/t0/pw_a115176.pdf.

Army Individual Test Battery. (1944). *Manual of directions and scoring.* Washington, DC: War Department, Adjutant General's Office.

Association of State and Provincial Psychology Boards. (2002). *ASPPB model regulations.* Montgomery, AL: Author.

Association of State and Provincial Psychology Boards. (2014a). *Competencies expected of psychologists at the point of licensure.* Retrieved from http:// c.ymcdn.com/sites/www.asppb.net/resource/resmgr/Guidelines/ ASPPB_Competencies_Expected_.pdf

Association of State and Provincial Psychology Boards. (2014b). *Disciplinary actions: 1974–2010.* Retrieved from http://c.ymcdn.com/sites/ www.asppb.net/resource/resmgr/dds/dds_historical_report_2010. pdf?hhSearchTerms=%22discipline+and+actions%22

Barlow, D. H. (Ed.). (2014). *Clinical handbook of psychological disorders: A step-by-step treatment manual* (5th ed.). New York, NY: Guilford Press. http://dx.doi.org/10.1093/oxfordhb/9780199328710.001.0001

Barnett, J. E. (2014). Sexual feelings and behaviors in the psychotherapy relationship: An ethics perspective. *Journal of Clinical Psychology, 70,* 170–181. http://dx.doi.org/10.1002/jclp.22068

Battistin, L., & Cagnin, A. (2010). Vascular cognitive disorder. A biological and clinical overview. *Neurochemical Research, 35,* 1933–1938. http://dx.doi.org/10.1007/s11064-010-0346-5

Beck, A. T. (1967). *Depression: Clinical, experimental, and theoretical aspects.* Philadelphia: University of Pennsylvania Press.

Beck A. T., Steer, R. A., & Brown G. K. (1996). *Manual for the Beck Depression Inventory-II.* San Antonio, TX: Psychological Corporation.

Beidel, D., Frueh, C., & Hersen, M. (Eds.). (2014). *Adult psychopathology and diagnosis* (7th ed.). New York, NY: Wiley.

Benedict, R. (1934). Anthropology and the abnormal. *The Journal of General Psychology, 10,* 59–82. http://dx.doi.org/10.1080/00221309. 1934.9917714

Bergin, A. E., & Garfield, S. L. (Eds.). (1971). *Handbook of psychotherapy and behavior change.* New York, NY: Wiley.

Bersoff, D. N. (2008). *Ethical conflicts in psychology* (4th ed.). Washington, DC: American Psychological Association.

Bersoff, D. N., DeMatteo, D., & Foster, E. E. (2012). *Assessment and testing.* In S. J. Knapp, (Ed.). *APA handbook of ethics in psychology* (pp. 45–74). Washington, DC: American Psychological Association.

Bhugra, D., Easter, A., Mallaris, Y., & Gupta, S. (2011). Clinical decision making in psychiatry by psychiatrists. *Acta Psychiatrica Scandinavica, 124*, 403–411. http://dx.doi.org/10.1111/j.1600-0447.2011.01737.x

Bhui, L., & Morgan, N. (2007). Effective psychotherapy in a racially and culturally diverse society. *Advances in Psychiatric Treatment, 13*, 187–193. http://dx.doi.org/10.1192/apt.bp.106.002295

Bolam v Friern Hospital Management Committee. (1957). Retrieved from http://oxcheps.new.ox.ac.uk/casebook/Resources/BOLAMV_1%20DOC.pdf

Borchard, B., Gnoth, A., & Schulz, W. (2003). Persönlichkeitsstörungen und "Psychopathy bei Sexualstraftätern im Maßregelvollzug—SKID–II- und PCL–R Befunde von Impulskontrollgestörten und Paraphilen [Personality disorders and "psychopathy" in sex offenders imprisoned in forensic-psychiatric hospitals—SKID–II- and PCL–R results in patients with impulse control disorder and paraphilia]. *Psychiatrische Praxis, 30*, 133–138. http://dx.doi.org/10.1055/s-2003-38607

Borsboom, D., Cramer, A. O. J., Schmittmann, V. D., Epskamp, S., & Waldorp, L. J. (2011). The small world of psychopathology. *PLoS ONE, 6*, e27407. http://dx.doi.org/10.1371/journal.pone.0027407

Bram, A., & Peebles, M. J. (2014). *Psychological testing that matters: Creating a road map for effective treatment.* Washington, DC: American Psychological Association. http://dx.doi.org/10.1037/14340-000

Bridges, N. A. (2001). Therapist's self-disclosure: Expanding the comfort zone. *Psychotherapy: Theory, Research, Practice, and Training, 38*, 21–30. http://dx.doi.org/10.1037/0033-3204.38.1.21

Brookfield, S. (1987). *Critical thinking: Challenging adults to explore alternative ways of thinking and acting.* San Francisco, CA: Jossey-Bass.

Brown, G. S., Jones, E. R., Betts, E., & Wu, J. (2003). Improving suicide risk assessment in a managed-care environment. *Crisis: The Journal of Crisis Intervention and Suicide Prevention, 24*, 49–55.

Brown, K., Keel, P. K., & Striegel, R. H. (2012). Feeding and eating conditions not elsewhere classified (NEC) in the *DSM–5. Psychiatric Annals, 42*, 421–425. http://dx.doi.org/10.3928/00485713-20121105-08

Butcher, J. N., Dahlstrom, W. G., Graham, J. R., Tellegen, A., & Kaemmer, B. (1989). *The Minnesota Multiphasic Personality Inventory—2 (MMPI–2): Manual for administration and scoring.* Minneapolis: University of Minnesota Press.

Butcher, J. N., Graham, J. R., & Ben-Porath, Y. S. (1995). Methodological problems and issues in MMPI, MMPI–2, and MMPI–A research. *Psychological Assessment, 7*, 320–329. http://dx.doi.org/10.1037/1040-3590.7.3.320

Butcher, J. N., Ones, D. S., & Cullen, M. (2006). Personnel screening with the MMPI–2. In J. N. Butcher (Ed.). *MMPI–2: A practitioner's guide* (pp. 381–406). Washington, DC: American Psychological Association

Butler, A., Chapman, J., Forman, E., & Beck, A. (2006). The empirical status of cognitive–behavioral therapy: A review of meta-analyses. *Clinical Psychology Review, 26,* 17–31. http://dx.doi.org/10.1016/j.cpr.2005.07.003

California Department of Corrections and Rehabilitation. (2010). *2010 adult institutions outcome evaluation report.* Retrieved from http://www.cdcr.ca.gov/adult_research_branch/research_documents/arb_fy0506_outcome_evaluation_report.pdf

Canadian Psychological Association. (2000). *Canadian code of ethics for psychologists* (3rd ed.). Ottawa, Ontario, Canada: Canadian Psychological Association. Retrieved from http://www.cpa.ca/docs/File/Ethics/cpa_code_2000_eng_jp_jan2014.pdf

Carkhuff, R. R. (2009). *The art of helping* (9th ed.). Amherst, MA: Human Resource Development Press.

Carlson, J. F., Geisinger, K. F., & Jonson, J. L. (Eds.). (2014). *The nineteenth mental measurements yearbook.* Lincoln: University of Nebraska Press

Carroll, L. (1865). *Alice's adventures in wonderland.* Retrieved from http://literature.org/authors/carroll-lewis/alices-adventures-in-wonderland/index.html

Castonguay, L. G., & Hill, C. E. (Eds.). (2012). *Transformation in psychotherapy: Corrective experiences across cognitive, behavioral, humanistic, and psychodynamic approaches.* Washington, DC: American Psychological Association. http://dx.doi.org/10.1037/13747-000

Cattell, R. B., Cattell, A. K., & Cattell, H. E. P. (2002). 16PF (5th ed.). San Antonio, TX: Pearson. Retrieved from http://www.pearsonclinical.com/psychology/products/100000483/16pf-fifth-edition.html#tab-details

Centers for Medicare and Medicaid Services. (2015a). *ICD–10–CM.* Retrieved from http://www.cms.gov/Medicare/Coding/ICD10/2015-ICD-10-CM-and-GEMs.html

Centers for Medicare and Medicaid Services. (2015b). *Mental health services.* Retrieved from http://www.cms.gov/Outreach-and-Education/Medicare-Learning-Network-MLN/MLNProducts/Downloads/Mental_Health_Services_ICN903195.pdf

Chambless, D. L., & Ollendick, T. H. (2001). Empirically supported psychological interventions: Controversies and evidence. *Annual Review of Psychology, 52,* 685–716. http://dx.doi.org/10.1146/annurev.psych.52.1.685

Clayton, C. (2007). *A guide to the lost art of critical thinking.* Lincoln, NE: iUniverse.

Colli, A., Tanzilli, A., Dimaggio, G., & Lingiardi, V. (2014). Patient personality and therapist response: An empirical investigation. *The American Journal of Psychiatry, 171,* 102–108. http://dx.doi.org/10.1176/appi.ajp.2013.13020224

Collins, K. A., & Clément, R. (2012). Language and prejudice: Direct and moderated effects. *Journal of Language and Social Psychology, 31,* 376–396. http://dx.doi.org/10.1177/0261927X12446611

Constantino, M. J., Arnkoff, D. B., Glass, C. R., Ametrano, R. M., & Smith, J. Z. (2011). Expectations. *Journal of Clinical Psychology, 67,* 184–192. http://dx.doi.org/10.1002/jclp.20754

Cornish, J., Schreier, B., Nadkarni, L., Metzger, L., & Rodolfa, E. (Eds.). (2010). *Handbook of multicultural competencies.* Hoboken, NJ: Wiley.

Costa, P. T., Jr., & McCrae, R. R. (2005). *NEO Personality Inventory—III (NEO-PI–III).* Odessa, FL: Psychological Assessment Resources.

Craig, R. J. (1999). Overview and current status of the Millon Clinical Multiaxial Inventory. *Journal of Personality Assessment, 72,* 390–406. http://dx.doi.org/10.1207/S15327752JP720305

Cressey, D. (2012, February 2). Informed consent on trial. *Nature, 482,* 16. Retrieved from http://www.nature.com/news/informed-consent-on-trial-1.9933

Cronbach, L. J., & Meehl, P. E. (1955). Construct validity in psychological tests. *Psychological Bulletin, 52,* 281–302. http://dx.doi.org/10.1037/h0040957

D'Zurilla, T. J., & Nezu, A. M. (1999). *Problem-solving therapy: A social competence approach to clinical intervention.* New York, NY: Springer.

Damasio, A. (1994). *Descartes' error: Emotion, reason, and the human brain.* New York, NY: Penguin Books.

Damasio, A. (2000). *The feeling of what happens: Body and emotion in the making of consciousness.* Boston, MA: Mariner Books.

Damasio, A. (2010). *Self comes to mind: Constructing the conscious brain.* New York, NY: Vintage Books.

Davies, M. F. (2003). Confirmatory bias in the evaluation of personality descriptions: Positive test strategies and output interference. *Journal of Personality and Social Psychology, 85,* 736–744. http://dx.doi.org/10.1037/0022-3514.85.4.736

Dawes, R. (1988). *Rational choice in an uncertain world.* San Diego, CA: Harcourt.

DeClue, G. (2013). Years of predicting dangerously. *Open Access Journal of Forensic Psychology, 5,* 16–28.

Deese, J., & Kaufman, R. A. (1957). Serial effects in recall of unorganized and sequentially organized verbal material. *Journal of Experimental Psychology, 54,* 180–187. http://dx.doi.org/10.1037/h0040536

Derlega, V. J., & Berg, J. H. (Eds.). (1987). *Self-disclosure: Theory, research, and therapy.* New York, NY: Plenum Press. http://dx.doi.org/10.1007/978-1-4899-3523-6

DeRubeis, R. J., Hollon, S. D., Amsterdam, J. D., Shelton, R. C., Young, P. R., Salomon, R. M., . . . Gallop, R. (2005). Cognitive therapy vs. medications in the treatment of moderate to severe depression. *Archives of General Psychiatry, 62,* 409–416. http://dx.doi.org/10.1001/archpsyc.62.4.409

Detrick, P., Chibnall, J. T., & Rosso, M. (2001). Minnesota Multiphasic Personality Inventory—2 in police officer selection: Normative data and relation to the Inwald Personality Inventory. *Professional Psychology: Research and Practice, 32,* 484–490. http://dx.doi.org/10.1037/0735-7028.32.5.484

Disease. (2014). In *Oxford Dictionary of American English*. Retrieved from http://www.oxforddictionaries.com/us/definition/american_english/disease

Duncan, B. L., Miller, S. D., Wampold, B. E., & Hubble, M. A. (Eds.). (2009). *The heart and soul of change: Delivering what works in therapy* (2nd ed.). Washington, DC: American Psychological Association.

Elliott, C. D. (2007). *Differential Abilities Scale—II*. San Antonio, TX: Pearson.

Ellis, A. (1973). *Reason and emotion in psychotherapy*. Secaucus, NJ: Lyle Stuart.

Evans, J. St. B. T. (1989). *Bias in human reasoning: Causes and consequences*. Hillsdale, N. J.: Erlbaum.

Evans, N., Gilpin, L., Holmes, G., Rafique, Z., & Yates, I. (2010). Power and status in groups. *Therapy Today, 21,* 26–29.

Facione, N. (2013). *Critical thinking: What it is and why it counts—2013 update*. Milbrae, CA: Measured Reasons and The California Academic Press. Retrieved from https://spu.edu/depts/health-sciences/grad/documents/CTbyFacione.pdf

Farber, B. A. (2006). *Self-disclosure in psychotherapy*. New York, NY: Guilford Press.

Festinger, L. (1957). *A theory of cognitive dissonance*. Evanston, IL: Row, Peterson.

Finn, S. E. (1996). *Manual for using the MMPI–2 as a therapeutic intervention*. Minneapolis: University of Minnesota Press.

First, M., Williams, J., Karg, R., & Spitzer, R. (2015). *Structured Clinical Interview for DSM–5 (SCID-5-CV), Clinician Version*. Arlington, VA: American Psychiatric Publishing.

Fischer, C. T. (2000). Collaborative, individualized assessment. *Journal of Personality Assessment, 74,* 2–14. http://dx.doi.org/10.1207/S15327752JPA740102

Fisher, C. B. (2003). *Decoding the ethics code: A practice guide for psychologists*. Thousand Oaks, CA: Sage.

Flanagan, D. P., & Harrison, P. L. (Eds.). (2005). *Contemporary intellectual assessment: Theories, tests, and issues* (2nd ed.). New York, NY: Guilford Press.

Frankl, V. E. (1963). *Man's search for meaning*. New York, NY: Pocket Books.

Gazzaniga, M. S. (2011). *Who's in charge? Free will and the science of the brain*. New York, NY: HarperCollins.

Goldberg, L. R. (1968). Simple models or simple processes? Some research on clinical judgments. *American Psychologist, 23,* 483–496. http://dx.doi.org/10.1037/h0026206

Gordijn, E., Finchilescu, G., Brix, L., Wijnants, N., & Koomen, W. (2008). The influence of prejudice and stereotypes on anticipated affect: Feelings about a potentially negative interaction with another ethnic group. *South African Journal of Psychology/Suid-Afrikaanse Tydskrif vir Sielkunde, 38*, 589–601. http://dx.doi.org/10.1177/008124630803800401

Gottschall, J. (2012). *The storytelling animal: How stories make us human.* New York, NY: Houghton Mifflin.

Gough, H. G. (1987). *California Psychological Inventory administrator's guide.* Palo Alto, CA: Consulting Psychologists Press.

Graham, J. R. (1990). *MMPI–2: Assessing personality and psychopathology* (2nd ed.). New York, NY: Oxford University Press.

Graham, J. R. (2000). *MMPI–2: Assessing personality and psychopathology* (3rd ed.). New York, NY: Oxford University Press.

Graybiel, A. M., & Smith, K. S. (2014). Good habits, bad habits. *Scientific American, 310*, 38–43. http://dx.doi.org/10.1038/scientificamerican 0614-38

Greenberg, L. S. (2002). *Emotion-focused therapy.* Washington, DC: American Psychological Association.

Greenberg, R. P., Constantino, M. J., & Bruce, N. (2006). Are patient expectations still relevant for psychotherapy process and outcome? *Clinical Psychology Review, 26*, 657–678. http://dx.doi.org/10.1016/ j.cpr.2005.03.002

Greenberg, S., & Shuman, D. (1997). Irreconcilable conflict between therapeutic and forensic roles. *Professional Psychology: Research and Practice, 28*, 50–57. http://dx.doi.org/10.1037/0735-7028.28.1.50

Greenberg, S., & Shuman, D. (2007). When worlds collide: Therapeutic and forensic roles. *Professional Psychology: Research and Practice, 38*, 129–132. http://dx.doi.org/10.1037/0735-7028.38.2.129

Greene, R. L. (2011). *The MMPI–2/MMPI–2–RF: An interpretive manual* (3rd ed.). Boston, MA: Allyn & Bacon.

Grove, W. M. (2005). Clinical versus statistical prediction: The contribution of Paul E. Meehl. *Journal of Clinical Psychology, 61*, 1233–1243. http://dx.doi.org/10.1002/jclp.20179

Grove, W. M., Zald, D. H., Lebow, B. S., Snitz, B. E., & Nelson, C. (2000). Clinical versus mechanical prediction: A meta-analysis. *Psychological Assessment, 12*, 19–30. http://dx.doi.org/10.1037/1040-3590.12.1.19

Hanson, R. K., & Bussière, M. T. (1998). Predicting relapse: A meta-analysis of sexual offender recidivism studies. *Journal of Consulting and Clinical Psychology, 66*, 348–362. http://dx.doi.org/10.1037/ 0022-006X.66.2.348

Harris, A. J. R., & Hanson, R. K. (2004). *Sex offender recidivism: A simple question* (Cat No. PS3-1/2004-3). Ottawa, Ontario, Canada: Public Works and Government Services.

Hatch-Maillette, M. A., Scalora, M. J., Huss, M. T., & Baumgartner, J. V. (2001). Criminal thinking patterns: Are child molesters unique? *International Journal of Offender Therapy and Comparative Criminology, 45*, 102–117. http://dx.doi.org/10.1177/0306624X01451007

Hathaway, S. R., & McKinley, J. C. (1942). *Manual for the Minnesota Multiphasic Personality Disorder.* Minneapolis: University of Minnesota Press.

Hayne, Y. M. (2003). Experiencing psychiatric diagnosis: Client perspectives on being named mentally ill. *Journal of Psychiatric and Mental Health Nursing, 10*, 722–729. http://dx.doi.org/10.1046/j.1365-2850.2003.00666.x

Health Insurance Portability and Accountability Act of 1996, Pub. L. 104–191, 1110 Stat. 1936.

Heller, J. (1961). *Catch-22.* New York, NY: Simon & Schuster.

Herbert, P. B., & Young, K. A. (2002). Tarasoff at twenty-five. *The Journal of the American Academy of Psychiatry and the Law, 30*, 275–281.

Hester, R., & Miller, W. (2002). *Handbook of alcoholism treatment approaches* (3rd ed.). Boston, MA: Pearson.

Hofmann, S., Asnaani, A., Vonk, I., Sawyer, A., & Fang, A. (2012). The efficacy of cognitive behavioral therapy: A review of meta-analyses. *Cognitive Therapy and Research, 36*, 427–440. http://dx.doi.org/10.1007/s10608-012-9476-1

Hofmann, S., & Smits, J. (2008). Cognitive–behavioral therapy for adult anxiety disorders: A meta-analysis of randomized placebo-controlled trials. *Journal of Clinical Psychiatry, 69*, 621–632. http://dx.doi.org/10.1037/a0016032

Hogg, M. A., & Williams, K. D. (2000). From I to we: Social identity and the collective self. *Group Dynamics: Theory, Research, and Practice, 4*, 81–97. http://dx.doi.org/10.1037/1089-2699.4.1.81

Holt, R. R. (1958). Clinical and statistical prediction; a reformulation and some new data. *Journal of Abnormal and Social Psychology, 56*, 1–12. http://dx.doi.org/10.1037/h0041045

Horvath, A. O., & Bedi, R. P. (2002). The alliance. In J. C. Norcross (Ed.), *Psychotherapy relationships that work* (pp. 37–69). New York, NY: Oxford University Press.

Hoyt, W. T., & Kerns, M.-D. (1999). Magnitude and moderators of bias in observer ratings: A meta-analysis. *Psychological Methods, 4*, 403–424. http://dx.doi.org/10.1037/1082-989X.4.4.403

Hulkower, R. (2010). The history of the Hippocratic oath: Outdated, inauthentic, and yet still relevant. *The Einstein Journal of Biology and Medicine, 25/26*, 41–44.

Hunsley, J. (2007). Training psychologists for evidence-based practice. *Canadian Psychology/Psychologie Canadienne, 48*, 32–42. http://dx.doi.org/10.1037/cp2007_1_32

Hunsley, J., & Lee, C. M. (2014). *Introduction to clinical psychology: An evidence based approach* (2nd ed.). New York, NY: Wiley.

Hurd, K., & Noller, P. (1988). Decoding deception: A look at the process. *Journal of Nonverbal Behavior, 12,* 217–233. http://dx.doi.org/10.1007/BF00987489

Jackson, J. C., Sinnott, P. L., Marx, B. P., Murdoch, M., Sayer, N. A., Alvarez, J. M., . . . Speroff, T. (2011). Variation in practices and attitudes of clinicians assessing PTSD-related disability among veterans. *Journal of Traumatic Stress, 24,* 609–613. http://dx.doi.org/10.1002/jts.20688

Jankowski, D. (2002). *A beginner's guide to the MCMI–III.* Washington, DC: American Psychological Association. http://dx.doi.org/10.1037/10446-000

Kahneman, D. (2011). *Thinking, fast and slow.* New York, NY: Farrar, Straus, & Giroux.

Kahneman, D., & Tversky, A. (1972). Subjective probability: A judgment of representativeness. *Cognitive Psychology, 3,* 430–454. http://dx.doi.org/10.1016/0010-0285(72)90016-3

Kaufman, A. S., & Kaufman, N. L. (1993). *Manual for the Kaufman Adolescent and Adult Intelligence Test (KAIT).* Circle Pines, MN: American Guidance Service.

Kaufman, A. S., & Lichtenberger, E. (2006). *Assessing adolescent and adult intelligence* (3rd ed.). Hoboken, NJ: Wiley.

Kelley, H. H. (1967). Attribution theory in social psychology. *Nebraska Symposium on Motivation, 15,* 192–238.

Kleck, R. E., & Strenta, A. (1980). Perceptions of the impact of negatively valued physical characteristics on social interaction. *Journal of Personality and Social Psychology, 39,* 861–873. http://dx.doi.org/10.1037/0022-3514.39.5.861

Krumholz, H. M. (2010). Informed consent to promote patient-centered care. *JAMA: Journal of the American Medical Association, 303,* 1190–1191. http://dx.doi.org/10.1001/jama.2010.309

Lambert, M. J. (Ed.). (2013). *Bergin and Garfield's handbook of psychotherapy and behavior change* (6th ed.). New York, NY: Wiley.

Lazarus, R. S., & Folkman, S. (1984). *Stress, appraisal, and coping.* New York, NY: Springer.

Lee, E. (2014). A therapist's self-disclosure and its impact on the therapy process in cross-cultural encounters: Disclosure of personal self, professional self, and/or cultural self? *Families in Society, 95,* 15–23. http://dx.doi.org/10.1606/1044-3894.2014.95.3

Lehrer, P. M., Woolfolk, R. L., Sime, W. E., & Barlow, D. H. (2008). *Principles and practice of stress management* (3rd ed.). New York, NY: Guilford.

Levak, R. W., Siegel, L., Nichols, D. S., & Stolberg, R. (2011). *Therapeutic feedback with the MMPI–2: A positive psychology approach.* New York, NY: Taylor & Francis.

Luhrmann, T. M. (2011). Hallucinations and sensory overrides. *Annual Review of Anthropology, 40*, 71–85. http://dx.doi.org/10.1146/annurev-anthro-081309-145819

Luhrmann, T. M., Padmavati, R., Tharoor, H., & Osei, A. (2014). Differences in voice-hearing experiences of people with psychosis in the USA, India, and Ghana: Interview-based study. *The British Journal of Psychiatry, 205*, 1–4.

Lyons, C., Hopley, P., & Horrocks, J. (2009). A decade of stigma and discrimination in mental health: Plus ça change, plus c'est la même chose (the more things change, the more they stay the same). *Journal of Psychiatric and Mental Health Nursing, 16*, 501–507. http://dx.doi.org/10.1111/j.1365-2850.2009.01390.x

Machiavelli, N. (2008). *Machiavelli's the Prince: Bold-faced principles on tactics, power, and politics* (R. McMahon, Ed., & W. K. Marriott, Trans.). New York, NY: Sterling. (Original work published 1532)

MacIntyre, A. (1998). *Short history of ethics: A history of moral philosophy from the Homeric Age to the 20th century* (2nd ed.). Notre Dame, IN: University of Notre Dame Press.

Mate, G. (2011). *When the body says no: Exploring the stress–disease connection.* New York, NY: Wiley.

Matuszak, J., & Piasecki, M. (2012, October 5). Interrater reliability in psychiatric diagnosis. *Psychiatric Times, 29*, 12–13. Retrieved from http://www.psychiatrictimes.com/dsm-5-0/inter-rater-reliability-psychiatric-diagnosis

McCrae, R. R., & Costa, P. T., Jr. (1987). Validation of the five-factor model of personality across instruments and observers. *Journal of Personality and Social Psychology, 52*, 81–90. http://dx.doi.org/10.1037/0022-3514.52.1.81

McDermott, P. A., Watkins, M. W., & Rhoad, A. M. (2014). Whose IQ is it?—Assessor bias variance in high-stakes psychological assessment. *Psychological Assessment, 26*(1), 207–214. http://dx.doi.org/10.1037/a0034832

McGrady, A., & Moss, D. (2013). *Pathways to illness, pathways to health.* New York, NY: Springer. http://dx.doi.org/10.1007/978-1-4419-1379-1

McGrew, K., & Flanagan, D. (1998). *The intelligence test desk reference: Gf-Gc cross-battery assessment.* New York, NY: Allyn & Bacon.

Medicare. (2013). *What Part B covers.* Retrieved from http://www.medicare.gov/what-medicare-covers/part-b/what-medicare-part-b-covers.html

Meehl, P. E. (1954). *Clinical versus statistical prediction: A theoretical analysis and a review of the evidence.* Minneapolis: University of Minnesota. http://dx.doi.org/10.1037/11281-000

Meehl, P. E. (1986). Causes and effects of my disturbing little book. *Journal of Personality Assessment, 50*, 370–375. http://dx.doi.org/10.1207/s15327752jpa5003_6

Mehr, K. E., Ladany, N., & Caskie, G. I. L. (2010). Trainee non-disclosure in supervision: What are they not telling you? *Counselling & Psychotherapy Research, 10*, 103–113. http://dx.doi.org/10.1080/14733141003712301

Meichenbaum, D. (1985). *Stress inoculation training.* New York, NY: Pergamon Press.

Meyer, G. J., Finn, S. E., Eyde, L. D., Kay, G. G., Moreland, K. L., Dies, R. R., . . . Reed, G. M. (2001). Psychological testing and psychological assessment. A review of evidence and issues. *American Psychologist, 56*, 128–165.

Miller, A. K., Rufino, K. A., Boccaccini, M. T., Jackson, R. L., & Murrie, D. C. (2011). On individual differences in person perception: Raters' personality traits relate to their psychopathy checklist-revised scoring tendencies. *Assessment, 18*, 253–260. http://dx.doi.org/10.1177/1073191111402460

Miller, J. (2009). The effects of expectations on experiences with psychotherapy. *Counselling Psychology Quarterly, 22*, 343–346. http://dx.doi.org/10.1080/09515070903265454

Miller, P. R., Dasher, R., Collins, R., Griffiths, P., & Brown, F. (2001). Inpatient diagnostic assessments: 1. Accuracy of structured vs. unstructured interviews. *Psychiatry Research, 105*, 255–264. http://dx.doi.org/10.1016/S0165-1781(01)00317-1

Millon, T. (1969). *Modern psychopathology: A biosocial approach to maladaptive learning and functioning.* Philadelphia, PA: W. B. Saunders.

Millon, T. (2006). *Millon Clinical Multiaxial Inventory—III* (3rd ed.). Minneapolis, MN: National Computer Systems.

Millon, T., & Bloom, C. (2008). *The Millon Inventories second edition: A practitioner's guide.* New York, NY: Guilford Press.

Mohr, D. C. (1995). Negative outcome in psychotherapy: A critical review. *Clinical Psychology: Science and Practice, 2*, 1–27. http://dx.doi.org/10.1111/j.1468-2850.1995.tb00022.x

Morey, L. C. (1991). *Personality Assessment Inventory professional manual.* Odessa, FL: Psychological Assessment Resources.

Motiuk, L., & Porporino, F. (1992). *The prevalence, nature, and severity of mental health problems among federal male inmates in Canadian penitentiaries.* Report no 24. Ottawa, Ontario, Canada: Correctional Services of Canada.

Murdock, B. B. (1962). The serial position effect of free recall. *Journal of Experimental Psychology, 64*, 482–488. http://dx.doi.org/10.1037/h0045106

Murphy, L. M., Geisinger, K. F., Carlson, J. F., & Spies, R. S. (2011). *Tests in print VIII.* Lincoln, NE: Buros Institute of Mental Measurements.

Murphy, M. C., Richeson, J. A., Shelton, J. N., Reinschmidt, M. L., & Bergsieker, H. B. (2013). Cognitive costs of contemporary prejudice.

Group Processes & Intergroup Relations, 16, 560–571. http://dx.doi.org/10.1177/1368430212468170

Murray, H. A. (1943). *Thematic Apperception Test manual.* Cambridge, MA: Harvard University Press.

Myers, N. L. (2011). Update: Schizophrenia across cultures. *Current Psychiatry Reports, 13,* 305–311. http://dx.doi.org/10.1007/s11920-011-0208-0

Naglieri, J. A., Das, J. P., & Goldstein, S. (2014). *Cognitive assessment system—Second edition.* Chicago, IL: Riverside.

Nagy, T. F. (2005). *Ethics in plain English: An illustrative casebook for psychologists* (2nd ed.). Washington, DC: American Psychological Association.

Nagy, T. F. (2011). *Essential ethics for psychologists: A primer for understanding and mastering core issues.* Washington, DC: American Psychological Association. http://dx.doi.org/10.1037/12345-000

National Center for Health Statistics. (2015). *International Classification of Diseases and Related Health Problems—10 Clinical Modification.* Washington DC: U.S. Government Printing Office. Retrieved from http://www.cdc.gov/nchs/icd/icd10cm.htm#icd2015

Neumann, C. S., & Hare, R. D. (2008). Psychopathic traits in a large community sample: Links to violence, alcohol use, and intelligence. *Journal of Consulting and Clinical Psychology, 76,* 893–899. http://dx.doi.org/10.1037/0022-006X.76.5.893

Nickerson, R. (1998). Confirmation bias: A ubiquitous phenomenon in many guises. *Review of General Psychology, 2,* 175–220. http://dx.doi.org/10.1037/1089-2680.2.2.175

Norcross, J. C. (2011a). *Conclusions and recommendations of the Inter-divisional (APA Divisions 12 & 29) Task Force of Evidence-Based Therapy Relationships.* Washington, DC: Society for the Advancement of Psychotherapy, American Psychological Association. Retrieved from http://www.divisionofpsychotherapy.org/continuing-education/task-force-on-evidence-based-therapy-relationships/conclusions-of-the-task-force/

Norcross, J. C. (Ed.). (2011b). *Psychotherapy relationships that work: Evidence-based responsiveness.* New York, NY: Oxford University Press. http://dx.doi.org/10.1093/acprof:oso/9780199737208.001.0001

Norcross, J. C., & Wampold, B. (2011). Evidence-based therapy relationships: research conclusions and clinical practices. *Psychotherapy, 48,* 98–102

Northup, S. (1855). *Twelve years a slave.* Baton Rouge: Louisiana State.

Ogles, B. M., Lambert, M. J., & Sawyer, J. D. (1995). Clinical significance of the National Institute of Mental Health Treatment of Depression Collaborative Research Program data. *Journal of Consulting and Clinical Psychology, 63,* 321–326. http://dx.doi.org/10.1037/0022-006X.63.2.321

Owen, J., Wong, J. Y., & Rodolfa, E. (2010). The relationship between clients' conformity to masculine norms and their perceptions of helpful therapist actions. *Journal of Counseling Psychology, 57,* 68–78. http://dx.doi.org/10.1037/a0017870

Oyebode, F. (2008). *Sims' symptoms in the mind.* New York, NY: Elsevier.

Pagoto, S. L., Spring, B., Coups, E. J., Mulvaney, S., Coutu, M. F., & Ozakinci, G. (2007). Barriers and facilitators of evidence-based practice perceived by behavioral science health professionals. *Journal of Clinical Psychology, 63,* 695–705. http://dx.doi.org/10.1002/jclp.20376

Paul, G. L. (1967). Strategy of outcome research in psychotherapy. *Journal of Consulting Psychology, 31,* 109–118. http://dx.doi.org/10.1037/h0024436

Pope, K. S. (2014). *10 fallacies in psychological assessment.* Retrieved from http://kspope.com/fallacies/assessment.php

Pope, K. S., & Vasquez, M. J. T. (2011). *Ethics in psychotherapy and counseling: A practical guide* (4th ed.). San Francisco, CA: Jossey-Bass/Wiley. http://dx.doi.org/10.1002/9781118001875

Proulx, T., & Inzlicht, M. (2012). The five "A"s of meaning maintenance: Finding meaning in the theories of sense-making. *Psychological Inquiry, 23,* 317–335.

Rabin, L. A., Barr, W. B., & Burton, L. A. (2005). Assessment practices of clinical neuropsychologists in the United States and Canada: A survey of INS, NAN, and APA Division 40 members. *Archives of Clinical Neuropsychology, 20,* 33–65. http://dx.doi.org/10.1016/j.acn.2004.02.005

Randolph, C. (2012). *Repeatable Battery for the Assessment of Neuropsychological Status Update (RBANS Update).* San Antonio, TX: Pearson.

Rapaport, D., Gill, M. M., & Schafer, R. (1974). *Diagnostic psychological testing.* New York, NY: International Universities Press.

Ready, R. E., & Veague, H. B. (2014). Training in psychological assessment: Current practices in clinical psychology programs. *Professional Psychology: Research and Practice, 45,* 278–282. http://dx.doi.org/10.1037/a0037439

Reed, G. (2013, May). *Improving the clinical utility of WHO's ICD–11: Concepts and evidence.* Presentation at the 166th Annual Meeting of the American Psychiatric Association, San Francisco, CA.

Rehm, L. P. (2010). *Depression: Advances in psychotherapy—Evidence-based practice.* Boston, MA: Hogrefe.

Reich, J., Zautra, A., & Hall, J. (2010). *Handbook of adult resilience.* New York, NY: Guilford Press.

Reitan, R. M., & Wolfson, D. (1993). *The Halstead-Reitan Neuropsychological Test Battery: Theory and clinical interpretation* (2nd ed.). Tucson, AZ: Neuropsychology Press

Richeson, J. A., & Shelton, J. N. (2007). Negotiating interracial interactions: Costs, consequences, and possibilities. *Current Directions in Psychological Science, 16,* 316–320. http://dx.doi.org/10.1111/j.1467-8721.2007.00528.x

Rodolfa, E., Greenberg, S., Hunsley, J., Smith-Zoeller, M., Cox, D., Sammons, M., Caro, C. (2013). A competency model for the practice of psychology. *Training and Education in Professional Psychology, 7*, 71–84.

Rogers, C. R. (1961). *On becoming a person.* Boston, MA: Houghton Mifflin.

Rogers, R. (2003). Forensic use and abuse of psychological tests: Multiscale inventories. *Journal of Psychiatric Practice, 9*, 316–320. http://dx.doi.org/10.1097/00131746-200307000-00008

Roid, G. (2003). *Stanford–Binet Intelligence Scales* (5th ed.). Itasca, IL: Riverside.

Rorschach, H. (1927). *Rorschach Test—Psychodiagnostic plates.* Cambridge, MA: Hogrefe.

Rowe, R., & Clark, T. (2008). A survey of psychiatrists' attitudes to schizoaffective disorder. *International Journal of Psychiatry in Clinical Practice, 12*, 25–30. http://dx.doi.org/10.1080/13651500701330916

Safran, J. D., Crocker, P., McMain, S., & Murray, P. (1990). Therapeutic alliance rupture as a therapy event for empirical investigation. *Psychotherapy: Theory, Research, Practice, and Training, 27*, 154–165. http://dx.doi.org/10.1037/0033-3204.27.2.154

Sattler, J. M., & Schaffer, J. B. (2014). Introduction to the behavioral, social, and clinical assessment of children. In J. M. Sattler (Ed.), *Assessment of children: Behavioral, social, and clinical foundations* (6th ed., pp. 1–46). La Mesa, CA: Jerome M. Sattler, Publisher.

Saulsman, L. M. (2011). Depression, anxiety, and the MCMI–III: Construct validity and diagnostic efficiency. *Journal of Personality Assessment, 93*, 76–83. http://dx.doi.org/10.1080/00223891.2010.528481

Schachter, S., & Singer, J. E. (1962). Cognitive, social, and physiological determinants of emotional state. *Psychological Review, 69*, 379–399. http://dx.doi.org/10.1037/h0046234

Schneider, W. J. (2013). *Misunderstanding regression to the mean* [Video file]. Retrieved from http://assessingpsyche.wordpress.com/2013/12/16/video-tutorial-misunderstanding-regression-to-the-mean/

Schrank, F. A., Mather, N., & McGrew, K. S. (2014). *Woodcock–Johnson III Tests of Cognitive Abilities.* Itasca, IL: Riverside

Schretlen, D. J., Munro, C. A., Anthony, J. C., & Pearlson, G. D. (2003). Examining the range of normal intraindividual variability in neuropsychological test performance. *Journal of the International Neuropsychological Society, 9*, 864–870.

Scriven, M., & Paul, R. (1987, July). *Statement defining critical thinking.* Paper presented at the 8th Annual International Conference on Critical Thinking and Education Reform, Sonoma State University, Rohnert Park, CA. Retrieved from http://www.criticalthinking.org/pages/defining-critical-thinking/766

Sellbom, M., Fischler, G. L., & Ben-Porath, Y. S. (2007). Identifying MMPI–2 predictors of police officer integrity and misconduct.

Criminal Justice and Behavior, 34, 985–1004. http://dx.doi.org/10.1177/0093854807301224

Serres, C. (2015, February 9). "Monumental" sex offender trial begins in St. Paul. *Minneapolis Star and Tribune.* Retrieved from http://www.startribune.com/trial-testing-minnesota-s-sex-offender-commitment-program-begins-in-st-paul/291267051/

Silver, N. (2012). *The signal and the noise: Why most predictions fail—but some don't.* New York, NY: The Penguin Press.

Smith, T. W., & Ruiz, J. M. (2002). Psychosocial influences on the development and course of coronary heart disease: Current status and implications for research and practice. *Journal of Consulting and Clinical Psychology, 70,* 548–568. http://dx.doi.org/10.1037/0022-006X.70.3.548

Snyder, C. R., & Elliott, T. R. (2005). Twenty-first century graduate education in clinical psychology: A four level matrix model. *Journal of Clinical Psychology, 61,* 1003–1054. http://dx.doi.org/10.1002/jclp.20164

Society of Clinical Psychology. (1993). *Task Force on Promotion and Dissemination of Psychological Procedure: Report.* Retrieved from http://www.div12.org/sites/default/files/InitialReportOfTheChamblessTaskForce.pdf

Society of Clinical Psychology. (2014). *Research-supported psychological treatments.* Retrieved from http://www.psychologicaltreatments.org

Sommers-Flanagan, R., & Sommers-Flanagan, J. (2007). *Becoming an ethical helping professional: Cultural and philosophical foundations.* Hoboken, NJ: Wiley.

Son, L. K., & Kornell, N. (2010). The virtues of ignorance. *Behavioural Processes, 83,* 207–212. http://dx.doi.org/10.1016/j.beproc.2009.12.005

Stansfeld, S. A., Fuhrer, R., Shipley, M. J., & Marmot, M. G. (2002). Psychological distress as a risk factor for coronary heart disease in the Whitehall II Study. *International Journal of Epidemiology, 31,* 248–255. http://dx.doi.org/10.1093/ije/31.1.248

Steger, M. F. (2012). Making meaning in life. *Psychological Inquiry, 23,* 381–385

Stiles, W. B., Hurst, R. M., Nelson-Gray, R., Hill, C. E., Greenberg, L. S., & Watson, J. C., . . . Hollon, S. D. (2006). What qualifies as research on which to judge effective practice? In J. C. Norcross, L. E. Beutler, & R. F. Levant (Eds.), *Evidence-based practices in mental health: Debate and dialogue on the fundamental questions* (pp. 57–131). Washington, DC: American Psychological Association.

Strack, S. (2008). *Essentials of the Millon Inventories Assessment* (3rd ed.). Hoboken, NJ: Wiley.

Strasburger, L. H., Gutheil, T. G., & Brodsky, B. A. (1997). On wearing two hats: Role conflict in serving as both psychotherapist and expert witness. *American Journal of Psychiatry, 154,* 448–456

Straus, S. E., & McAlister, F. A. (2000). Evidence-based medicine: A commentary on common criticisms. *Canadian Medical Association Journal, 163,* 837–841.

Stuart, R. B. (1980). *Helping couples change: A social learning approach to marital therapy.* New York, NY: Guilford Press.

Sue, D., & Sue, D. (2003). *Counseling the culturally diverse: Theory and practice* (4th ed.). New York, NY: Wiley.

Sue, D., & Torino, G. (2005). Racial-cultural competence: awareness, knowledge, and skills. In R. T. Carter (Ed.), *Handbook of racial-cultural psychology and counseling: Training and practice* (Vol. 2, pp. 3–18). Hoboken, NJ: Wiley.

Szasz, T. S. (1961). *The myth of mental illness.* New York, NY: Harper & Row.

Tajfel, H., & Turner, J. C. (1986). The social identity theory of intergroup behavior. In S. Worchel & W. Austin (Eds.), *Psychology of intergroup relations* (2nd ed., pp. 7–24). Chicago, IL: Nelson-Hall.

Tarasoff v. The Regents of the University of California, 551 P.2d 334 (1976).

Tavris, C. (1989). *Anger: The misunderstood emotion.* New York, NY: Simon & Schuster.

Tavris, C., & Aronson, E. (2007). *Mistakes were made (but not by me): Why we justify foolish beliefs, bad decisions, and hurtful acts.* San Diego, CA: Harcourt.

Teixeira, R., & Halpin, J. (2013). *Building an all-in nation: A view from the American public.* Center for American Progress. Retrieved from http://www.americanprogress.org/issues/race/report/2013/10/22/77665/building-an-all-in-nation/

Tellegen, A., Ben-Porath, Y. S., McNulty, J. L., Arbisi, P. A., Graham, J. R., & Kaemmer, B. (2003). *MMPI–2 Restructured Clinical (RC) Scales: Development, validation, and interpretation.* Minneapolis: University of Minnesota Press.

Tracey, T. J., Lichtenberg, J. W., Goodyear, R. K., Claiborn, C. D., & Wampold, B. E. (2003). Concept mapping of therapeutic common factors. *Psychotherapy Research, 13,* 401–413. http://dx.doi.org/10.1093/ptr/kpg041

Truax, C. B., & Carkhuff, R. R. (1967). *Toward effective counseling and psychotherapy.* New York, NY: Aldine

Truax, C. B., & Carkhuff, R. R. (2007). *Toward effective counseling and psychotherapy: Training and practice.* Piscataway, NJ: Transaction.

Trull, T. (2005). *Clinical psychology* (7th ed.). Belmont, CA: Thomson Wadsworth.

Turner, J. S., & Leach, D. J. (2012). Behavioural activation therapy: Theory, concepts, and techniques. *Behaviour Change, 29,* 77–96. http://dx.doi.org/10.1017/bec.2012.3

Tyrer, P., Crawford, M., Mulder, R., Blashfield, R., Farnam, A., Fossati, A., . . . Reed, G. (2011). The rationale for the reclassification of personality disorder in the 11th revision of the *International Classification of Diseases (ICD–11)*. *Personality and Mental Health, 5,* 246–259.

Uebel, T. (2011). Vienna circle. In E. N. Zalta (Ed.), *The Stanford encyclopedia of philosophy.* Retrieved from http://plato.stanford.edu/entries/vienna-circle/#VieCirHis

U.S. Department of Health and Human Services. (2014). *Health information privacy.* Retrieved from http://www.hhs.gov/ocr/privacy/

U.S. Department of Health and Human Services. (2015). *Summary of the HIPAA privacy rule.* Retrieved from http://www.hhs.gov/ocr/privacy/hipaa/understanding/summary/index.html

Van Horne, B. A. (2004). Psychology licensing board disciplinary actions: The realities. *Professional Psychology: Research and Practice, 35,* 170–178. http://dx.doi.org/10.1037/0735-7028.35.2.170

Walfish, S., Vance, D., & Fabricatore, A. N. (2007). Psychological evaluation of bariatric surgery applicants: Procedures and reasons for delay or denial of surgery. *Obesity Surgery, 17,* 1578–1583. http://dx.doi.org/10.1007/s11695-007-9274-0

Wechsler, D. (2008). *Wechsler Adult Intelligence Scale—IV technical and interpretive manual.* San Antonio, TX: Pearson.

Wechsler, D. (2009). *Wechsler Memory Scales—Fourth Edition (WMS–IV).* San Antonio, TX: Pearson.

Wechsler, D. (2014). *Wechsler Intelligence Scale for Children—V technical and interpretive manual.* San Antonio, TX: Pearson.

Weinberg, J. R. (2001). *An examination of logical positivism.* London, England: Routledge.

Weiner, B. (1986). *An attribution theory of motivation and emotion.* New York, NY: Springer-Verlag. http://dx.doi.org/10.1007/978-1-4612-4948-1

Weiner, I. B. (2013). Psychological assessment is here to stay. *Archives of Assessment Psychology, 3,* 11–21.

Weston, D., & Morrison, K. (2001). A multidimensional meta-analysis of treatments for depression, panic, and generalized anxiety disorder: an empirical examination of the status of empirically supported therapies. *Journal of Consulting and Clinical Psychology, 69,* 875–899.

White, K., Nielson, W., Harth, M., Ostbye, T., Speechley, M. (2002). Chronic widespread musculoskeletal pain with or without fibromyalgia: psychological distress in a representative community adult sample. *The Journal of Rheumatology, 29,* 588–594.

Wiener, C., Fauci, A., Braunwald, E., Kasper, D., & Hauser, S. (2012). *Harrison's principles of internal medicine: Self-assessment and board review* (18th ed.). New York, NY: McGraw-Hill.

Wiggins, J. S. (Ed.). (1996). *The five-factor model of personality: Theoretical perspectives.* New York, NY: Guilford Press.

Wood, J. M., Nezworski, M. T., Lilienfeld, S. O., & Garb, H. N. (2003). *What's wrong with the Rorschach? Science confronts the controversial inkblot test.* New York, NY: Jossey-Bass.

Woody, S., Detweiler-Bedell, B., Teachman, B., & O'Hearn, T. (2004). *Treatment planning in psychotherapy: Taking the guesswork out of clinical care*. New York, NY: Guilford Press.

World Health Organization. (1949). *International statistical classification of diseases, injuries, and causes of death, 6th revision*. Geneva, Switzerland: Author.

World Health Organization. (1993). *ICD–10 classification of mental and behavioural disorders (blue book)*. Geneva, Switzerland: Author. Retrieved from http://www.who.int/classifications/icd/en/bluebook.pdf

World Health Organization. (2016). *International Statistical Classification of Diseases and Related Health Problems—10*. Geneva, Switzerland: Author. Retrieved from http://www.who.int/classifications/icd/en/

Yang, M., Wong, S. C. P., & Coid, J. (2010). The efficacy of violence prediction: A meta-analytic comparison of nine risk assessment tools. *Psychological Bulletin, 136*, 740–767. http://dx.doi.org/10.1037/a0020473

Zander, T. K. (2005). Civil commitment without psychosis: The law's reliance on the weakest links in psychodiagnosis. *The Journal of Sexual Offender Civil Commitment, Science and the Law, 1*, 17–82.

Zubin, J. (1956). Clinical versus actuarial prediction: A pseudo-problem. In N. Sanford, C. C. McArthur, J. Zubin, L. G. Humphreys, & P. E. Meehl (Eds.), *Proceedings of the Conference on Testing Problems* (pp. 625–637). Princeton, NJ: Educational Testing Service.

Index

About the Authors

Jack Schaffer, PhD, spent 17 years in independent practice and 16 years as faculty in two medical schools and a professional school. His private practice specialized in clinical and neuropsychological assessments and psychotherapy with adults and families. He received his doctorate in clinical psychology from The University of North Dakota and is certified by the American Board of Professional Psychology in clinical psychology and clinical health psychology. He is a fellow and past president of the Association of State and Provincial Psychology Boards and a past chair of the State of Minnesota Board of Psychology. He currently serves on the American Psychological Association's Commission on Accreditation. Dr. Schaffer's professional interests include psychological assessment, defining and assessing professional competence, and ethical and legal issues. He enjoys woodworking, bicycling, and spending time with his wife, his two children, and four grandchildren.

Emil Rodolfa, PhD, is a professor of psychology at Alliant International University's California School of Professional Psychology (CSPP) in Sacramento. He received his doctorate from Texas A&M University and was training director and director of the University of California Counseling and Psychological Services prior to joining the faculty at CSPP. He is the founding editor of *Training and Education in Professional Psychology* and was Associate Editor of *Professional Psychology Research and Practice*. Dr. Rodolfa is a fellow of the American Psychological Association, a fellow and past president of the Association of State and Provincial Psychology Boards, a Board Member Emeritus and past chair of the Association of Psychology Postdoctoral and Internship Centers, and a past president of the State of California Board of Psychology. His professional interests include defining and assessing professional competence, ethical and legal issues, supervision and training, college student mental health, and the assessment and treatment of anxiety and depression. He enjoys spending time with his family, playing horseshoes and BBQing (some might call it grilling) at his cabin in the mountains.